SPORT & REMEDIAL MASSAGE THERAPY

SPORT & REMEDIAL MASSAGE THERAPY

MEL CASH

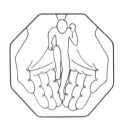

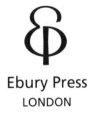

Ebury Press
LONDON

First published in 1996

11

First published in the United Kingdom in 1996 by
Ebury Press
an imprint of Random House
20 Vauxhall Bridge Road, London SW1V 2SA

Random House Australia (Pty) Limited,
20 Alfred Street, Milsons Point, Sydney,
New South Wales 2061, Australia.

Random House New Zealand Limited,
18 Poland Road, Glenfield,
Auckland 10, New Zealand.

Random House (Pty) Limited,
Endulini, 5a Jubilee Rd, Parktown 2193, South Africa.

The Random House Group Limited Reg. No. 954009

ISBN 0 09 180956 8

Design & make-up: Roger Walker

Printed and bound in Great Britain by
Scotprint, Haddington, Scotland

Any information given in this book is not intended to be taken as a replacement for medical advice. Any person with a condition requiring medical attention should consult a qualified practitioner.

Contents

Acknowledgements

Advisors
ALASTAIR GREETHAM, MCSP, Chartered Physiotherapist
ALEX FUGALLO, LLB (Hons), B.Sc. (Hons), DO, ND

Photography

Photographer	GAVIN COTTRELL
Director	ALEX FUGALLO
Therapists	MEL CASH
	RICK MEDLOCK
Models	GARY REES
	CHRISTINA ROBILLIARD
	ALEX FUGALLO

Anatomical Drawings
DIANE MAINZER

My knowledge has developed through experience and I am therefore grateful to every therapist I have worked with or been treated by; and to every patient I have treated and every student I have taught.

Special thanks go to my colleague Rick Medlock, who has freely shared his clinical knowledge and experience with me for over ten years.

Introduction

Massage is a natural therapy, which has probably been in use since the origins of mankind. It remained the principal method of treating most musculoskeletal problems for many thousands of years, and it was only in the last hundred years or so that this practice began to change.

Massage does have some treatment limitations, and to overcome these modern science has developed new techniques and technology. Today orthodox medicine, as it strives to make continual advances, has to some extent swept massage aside in favour of newer treatment methods. But massage has many benefits, both physical and psychological. Although new techniques and technology may be able to achieve some of these benefits, none can reproduce all of them. Massage works on many levels, and it is the unique way in which it combines the various benefits to suit the individual that makes it such a versatile and effective treatment method.

In my own practice I have seen many patients with problems that have not been improved by other courses of therapy (physiotherapy, osteopathy, chiropractic and even surgery). In many of these cases massage has quickly and effectively resolved the problem, proving that it is often the best treatment method. And, in a complementary role with other therapies, massage can greatly speed recovery because of its wide-ranging benefits.

Minor injury is by far the most common musculoskeletal problem, but as modern medicine puts effort into developing ways of treating increasingly serious conditions, minor everyday injuries are becoming less adequately dealt with, although they can still be extremely painful and may seriously affect a person's occupation, sport or quality of life. Furthermore, if not treated properly at an early stage, a minor injury can sometimes lead to a more serious condition in the long term. Massage can treat the majority of such minor problems quickly and effectively, and it therefore needs be made more readily available to the general public.

Injury prevention is another area where the importance of massage should not be underestimated. Modern scientific understanding has developed an 'advice'-centred approach to injury prevention, based on assessment and exercise, and it is not seen as a 'treatable' situation. Massage is the only actual treatment that can be applied specifically to help prevent injury. This is not only true in a sports context, but also in terms of posture and other forms of stress.

Although many medical practitioners do understand the value of massage, they often find that they have insufficient time to do it properly.

And, as a skill, massage demands considerable regular practice to become proficient enough to achieve good results. For this reason complementary therapists should be encouraged, through good training, to concentrate on this vital area of treatment. There is a need for a level of therapy that can effectively treat and prevent minor problems and safely refer potentially serious conditions to a medical practitioner.

The aim of this book is to help create a greater awareness and understanding of the uses of massage, by bringing its ancient skills up-to-date with a modern understanding of how the body both functions and dysfunctions. In this way it is hoped that massage will once again be recognized as a major component in musculoskeletal health care.

About this book

This book is intended for people in different countries within a wide range of disciplines: doctors, physiotherapists, osteopaths, massage therapists, as well as sports coaches and trainers. This makes it difficult to use terms that will satisfy all readers. For the sake of simplicity, the term 'therapist' has been used to refer to the person giving the massage treatment and the term 'patient' to refer to the person receiving the treatment.

Clinical job titles and professional demarcation lines may also vary in certain countries and may slightly affect the text in some places.

Although, wherever possible, I have tried to avoid the situation, it has been necessary to use the masculine form on occasions (sports*men*, for example). I apologize to female readers, and the text of course refers throughout to both men and women, unless otherwise stated.

Student's note: Those who are new to this subject should become familiar with the content of the appendices before reading beyond Chapter 9.

1 Some Practicalities

Massage is a natural therapy, which can be practised anywhere and without any equipment, if necessary. But to work professionally it is essential to consider how to create the right environment to achieve the best results for the patient, with the least fatigue and stress on the therapist.

The most important factor effecting good results is the degree of relaxation of the patient. This is not just achieved by attending to physical comfort, for he (or she) also has to feel comfortable with the therapist and confident that he will get good treatment. Therapists sometimes find that the clinical white tunic does not convey the relaxed, friendly approach that puts people at ease. It is also important that the therapist feels comfortable as he (or she) works, and for these reasons many tend to wear a smart but casual uniform.

This approach should also be reflected in the treatment room, which may not benefit from appearing too clinical. It must still, however, look professional, to put the client at their ease. Charts of the muscular and skeletal systems should be hung on the wall. These can be used to point out the structures involved in any problem that the patient may have. This can help him visualize the problem and can be a strong psychological aid to recovery.

The treatment room should be warm, quiet and well ventilated. Warmth is the most important of these, as it is not possible to relax well if the muscles are cold. But massage is just as vital at sports venues and other locations as it is in a specially prepared room and the therapist must be able to work wherever he is: track-side, road-side, in a changing room, etc. Wherever the therapist works it is important to try to create a relaxing environment.

Treatment couch

The most important piece of equipment that a therapist should have is a treatment couch (plinth). This allows him to move freely around the patient and work from different directions, and enables the efficient use of body weight at all times. A couch should have a face hole, so that when the patient is lying in the prone position (face down), the neck is in a neutral, relaxed position. Where a couch is not available it is best

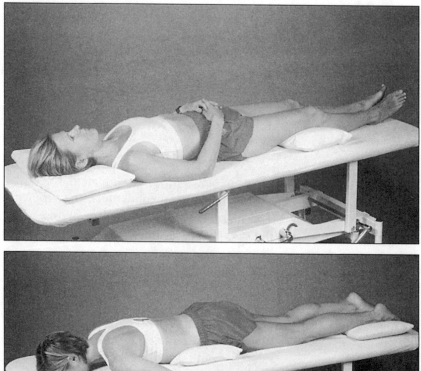

Lying in the supine position with cushions under the head and knees to increase relaxation.

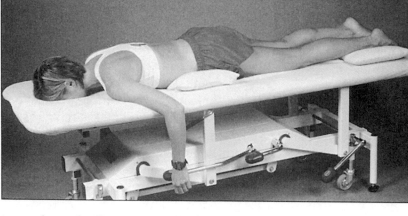

Lying in the prone position with cushions under the hips and ankles to increase relaxation.

to work on the floor (covered with a blanket for comfort). Although very effective treatment can be given on the floor, it is not ideal for the therapist, as it is uncomfortable on the knees and can cause back problems. A bed should not be used as the patient will only sink into it as pressure is applied, and it is also bad for the therapist's lower back.

Ideally, a treatment couch should have a mechanical height adjustment so that it can be raised or lowered during treatment, depending on the size of the client, the part being treated and the amount of pressure that needs to be applied. The couch height may need adjusting several times during one treatment to achieve the best results with the least effort and stress to the therapist. When working at other venues, a portable couch is usually needed. These come in a variety of fixed heights and it is best to choose one that comes up to the therapist's mid-thigh. Any couch that cannot be adjusted during treatment will mean that there has to be some compromise in the most efficient use of body weight, and over a long period of time this could lead to the therapist experiencing back problems himself. The therapist should set a good example and take remedial steps (exercise) to prevent this.

Cushions

It is important to have a variety of cushions available to support parts of the body. When a patient is in the prone position, placing a cushion under the ankles will shorten and relax the hamstrings and calf muscles and reduce the possibility of cramp occurring in the foot. In the supine position (lying face up), a cushion under the neck and one under the knees will create a more relaxed position.

People with chronic lower back problems may find it more comfortable to have cushions under the hips (lying prone) and this is usually a better position for treatment too. In cases of chronic neck tension, placing a cushion under the shoulders (prone) so that the neck rests in flexion may also be very helpful. Where there is acute inflammation affecting a distal part of a limb, cushions can support it in an elevated position to assist lymphatic drainage. Cushions may be used in many applications to support and provide comfort.

Towels

Towels (or similar) should be used to keep the patient covered, with only the area being treated left exposed. This has both physical and psychological benefits. It keeps the body warm, so aiding relaxation, which is particularly important after an area has been treated. This will maintain the heat generated by the massage and prevent the chilling effect of any evaporating oil. Towels also give the client the feeling of comfort and security that will further help general relaxation. When working closely in the groin or chest areas (in women), a towel can create a psychological security barrier, putting the client more at ease. So even in warm conditions it is important to keep the patient properly covered.

The student needs to use common sense and practice to develop a good, confident towel procedure. The whole body should be covered as soon as the patient lies down, and then each area should be uncovered as it is treated. When the patient rolls over, the towel can be held down along one side (away from the direction of the roll) so that he continually remains covered. Tucking the edge of the towel under any clothing that the patient wears will prevent oil stains getting on them, but too much tucking-in can be very obtrusive to the patient, so this technique should be practised.

For demonstration purposes the photographs in this book show the patient without *the correct covering.*

Lubricants

All the main techniques used in massage require a lubricant of some sort. Oil is the lubricant most commonly used, but there are liquefying creams and fine powders that can also work well. Some products may contain ingredients that cause adverse skin reactions (on the patient or the therapist's hands) and care should be taken when selecting a product. As some oil may be absorbed through the skin into the blood circulation, it is important when treating competitive sportsmen that there are no banned substances present in it.

A lubricant is necessary to allow the therapist's hands to slide over the skin without causing surface friction. If too little is used, especially on people with a lot of body hair, it could leave the skin feeling sore, and by irritating the hair follicles may cause these to become inflamed (folliculitis) and create a rash. As massage is at times extremely deep, it is important not to apply too much oil either, as this could prevent good control. It is best to apply it little and often, and the amount should vary depending on the techniques being used and the nature of the patient's skin. The best way to do this is to have the oil (or other lubricant) close by in a container that requires only one hand to operate it, so that the other hand can stay in contact with the patient.

2 The Effects of Massage

General circulation

All the cells of the body need a good supply of blood, which contains all the ingredients needed for their growth, repair and nutrition. The cells also need to eliminate the waste materials that arise from the production of energy, and debris from any tissue damage or inflammation. The stroking techniques of massage have a pumping effect, which stimulates the circulation of blood and so increases both the supply and removal of substances on a cellular level. As well as being beneficial to local tissues, the general circulatory stimulation can help improve the health or recovery of most other systems of the body.

The blood is pumped from the heart through arteries, which grow smaller and smaller as they diverge and become tiny arterioles on a cellular level. The blood is drawn back towards the heart through veins, which begin with tiny capillaries that merge with the arterioles. These grow larger and larger as they converge towards the heart. As the arteries narrow they maintain high pressure in the vessels, but that pressure is much lower in the veins as they become wider. The difference in pressure, where the arterioles and capillaries meet, enables the cells to absorb the substances needed from the arterial blood supply and the venous return to absorb the substances that need to be removed.

In the limbs, particularly the lower legs, the weaker pressure in the veins can mean that blood-flow becomes very slow. And due to the force of gravity there may even be a risk of a dangerous back-flow. To prevent this, the veins contain non-return valves at regular intervals along their length.

To stimulate circulation with massage it is necessary to apply pressure using long strokes in the same direction as the venous return (towards the heart). As the blood is pushed up the vein, the vacuum created behind it will immediately be filled by fresh arterial blood. Pressure strokes should never be applied in the opposite direction, as this would force the blood against the non-return valves, causing damage to them and to the vessel walls. Although the strokes work against the arterial flow, these vessels are not adversely affected due to their strong pressure and because they generally run much more deeply through the body.

Even passive pressure and squeezing techniques have a pumping effect on circulation. The pressure forces the blood out of the vessels in one direction only, towards the heart, because of the non-return valves. When pressure is released, the vessels re-fill from the arterial supply.

Micro circulation

The walls of the blood vessels need to be soft and pliable so that they can assist the pumping action and allow filtration and absorption through them. As a massage stroke forces blood through the capillaries and arterioles it has a stretching effect on the vessel walls, which can help increase their size, capacity and function.

Lymphatic flow

Lymphatic vessels are not part of the circulatory system as they begin at a cellular level and travel in one direction only, towards the heart. They absorb excess interstitial fluid and return it to the venous system via lymph nodes, which filter out any toxins. The demands on the lymphatic system are greatest when there is an increase in the amount of interstitial fluid, which usually occurs through tissue injury, following hard exercise or as a result of other medical conditions.

As lymph vessels are not part of the pumped circulatory system, there is no intrinsic pressure to move the fluids through them. The motive force comes through muscle contraction, which is often limited when injury is involved, and gravity can also have a strong negative effect, especially in the lower leg.

The lymph vessels generally run parallel to the veins, and massage strokes greatly stimulate the flow through both of them at the same time.

Interstitial permeability

The movement and containment of all bodily fluids (not just the blood) are controlled by the various tissues with which they are in contact. In most cases these tissues have tiny pores that allow certain chemicals to pass through while others are held back. If these structures become thick and fibrous, the pores may close and the flow of interstitial fluid will suffer.

The mechanical effect of forcing fluids through the tissues by applying strong massage strokes can help to open these pores and improve this situation.

Scar tissue

When tissue damage occurs, some bleeding will take place and will develop into scar tissue, which is a vital part of the initial healing process. However, very often too much bleeding occurs, which can lead to excessive amounts of scar tissue forming. And with chronic inflammation more scar tissue will continually form as the condition persists. Scar tissue hardens over time and can eventually, in extreme cases, calcify and become just as hard as bone.

Friction massage techniques in the post-acute or chronic stages will prevent excessive scar tissue formation by stopping these cells from binding together. Where scar tissue has formed, friction can break it down into smaller particles, which can be digested by phagocyte cells and absorbed into the lymph vessels.

Adhesions and fibrous tissue

It is the adhesions and fibrous tissue created by the scar tissue that cause the real problem in tissue function. In the early stages, scar tissue is quite sticky and can adhere fibres together. For a muscle to function, the fibres need to be able to glide smoothly alongside one another, but when stuck together they cannot do this and the affected area will not function (contract or stretch). Over time, a local area of muscle fibres can mat together into a hard lump or knot.

The non-contractile soft tissues can also be affected by fibrous adhesion forming from scar tissue, which will make them thick and less pliable. Adhesions can also form between different structures, such as between a ligament and tendon or a muscle and bone. This can lead to a significant restriction in movement and function.

Transverse strokes and friction techniques can break down the adhesions by literally tearing the adhesive bonds apart. Once the fibres are separated they are able to function again. Although this does cause pain, it does not cause any actual damage because the adhesions themselves contain no blood vessels. If done too heavily or on tissue that is in an early stage of repair, further damage can be caused (see Chapter 3).

When a large fibrous knot of compacted tissue has formed there may be little or no circulation running through it and therefore a natural healing process cannot take place. Friction can loosen the knot and allow blood to flow more easily through it, which will stimulate healing and continue the breakdown process. Often a large knot will appear to have reduced by only 10 per cent at the end of a massage session, but when palpated four or five days later it may appear to have reduced by a further 20 or 30 per cent.

Tissue flexibility

Massage is able to stretch specific localized areas of tissue in a way that may not be possible with functional exercise. Regardless of functional range, deep longitudinal stroking can stretch the tissues by drawing them apart and in all possible directions. Even when stretching is not the specific aim of treatment, patients invariably find that they have greater range and freedom of movement after treatment due to the stretching effect of longitudinal stroking.

Nervous system

Massage can affect the nervous system in several ways. It stimulates the nerve receptors in the tissues, which control tissue tension. On a sensory level, the mechano-receptors that respond to touch, pressure, warmth and so on are also stimulated. These can all have a reflex effect, which leads to further relaxation of the tissues and a reduction in pain.

Tension in the soft tissues may reduce output from the mechano-receptors, which can cause over-activity in the sympathetic nervous system. By releasing this tension, massage can restore the balance and stimulate the parasympathetic system (which is why a patient's stomach will often make a rumbling sound – the parasympathetic system stimulates digestion). This can have a positive effect on both minor and sometimes quite major medical conditions, such as high blood pressure, migraine, insomnia and digestive disorders.

In more general terms, the total sensory input to the central nervous system affects overall tension throughout the body. This is why non-physical stress (emotional, etc.) can lead to physical symptoms, such as headaches, digestive problems and muscular discomfort. Massage works on so many levels, all of which aim to reduce the symptoms that cause negative sensory input and to increase the positive input. This accounts for the general feeling of well-being that patients usually feel after treatment.

3 Contraindications to Massage

Contraindications (as opposed to indications) relate to conditions where treatment (in this case massage) must not be applied, because it could increase the symptoms or create other problems. In most cases this is a local condition and only the affected area has to be avoided, while treatment to other areas may be very beneficial. There are also some general contraindications, which prevent any massage at all from being given.

Massage has proved over the centuries to be a very safe therapy. It is non-invasive as it does not penetrate the body, and as the skin forms such a good protective barrier, massage can only work with, and not change, the body's natural chemistry. Massage is also a very instant and direct form of treatment; if it is doing any harm it will usually be very painful at the time and the therapist can stop immediately. There are, however, some potential dangers and the therapist must always be diligent.

It is possible to over-treat an otherwise safe condition by applying too much deep stroking and friction, and inevitably this does happen from time to time. The consequences are not serious, however, and the worst that usually results is a small inflammation, which should clear up in a day or two. When treating some chronic conditions, a small inflammation is sometimes caused intentionally to act as a catalyst that triggers the chemistry involved in the healing process.

The first points considered here are the conditions that may initially present themselves as minor soft tissue problems, but which are in fact contraindicated. Most of these can be treated with massage in the post-acute phase and/or in conjunction with other medical treatment and they are therefore dealt with in more detail elsewhere in this book.

Acute soft tissue inflammation

This is by far the most common contraindication to face the massage therapist, and methods of treatment in the acute and post-acute phases are explained in Chapter 14. Acute inflammation can occur to any of the soft tissues (or organs):

- Muscles
- Tendons
- Ligaments

- Bursae
- Synovial capsule
- Inter-vertebral discs
- Periosteum, etc.

The most common causes are trauma and over-use, although some medical conditions can cause very similar symptoms:

- Strain (over-use, usually of muscle or tendon)
- Sprain (trauma to ligaments)
- Impact
- Pressure
- Rubbing, etc.

The common symptoms are:

- Pain and dysfunction in the affected area
- Heat and redness observed in the overlying skin
- Swelling local to the injury
- Frequently an obvious cause (trauma)

Where the affected tissues are more superficial, the symptoms are usually easy to identify. But where inflammation occurs to deep tissues, or where damage is contained within a compartment (intramuscular haematoma), the symptoms may not be visible, only palpable. Areas deep in the tissues may feel harder and more dense, and when pressed may cause a sharp pain. This could indicate an acute problem that must be avoided; however, non-acute and chronic problems will also feel harder and cause pain when pressed. In these situations deep friction, though painful, is very effective. It is therefore necessary to be able to differentiate between the two conditions.

With experience, the therapist can feel the subtle textural difference between the acute condition, which should not be treated, and the non-acute, which can be. The acute tends to feel softer, with a less clearly defined border, than the non-acute. This is, of course, a rather vague and subjective description and should not be relied upon on its own.

The patient's response to pain is also an indicator of the situation. Although considerable pain is often caused when applying deep techniques, the patient usually finds this tolerable (sometimes described as a 'good pain'). This is because, although fibrous adhesions are being torn apart, no actual tissue damage is being caused. If the tissues are acutely inflamed and the technique is causing further damage, the pain will feel intolerable and the patient will contract the muscles or attempt to move away.

10-second rule of thumb Another way to test for acute inflammation is by applying enough pressure to the area to cause mild discomfort. Maintain this fixed pressure for up to 10 seconds, during which time the patient is asked if the discomfort increases or decreases. If it increases this suggests that the tissues are in an acute state; if it decreases it is safe to treat.

Open wounds

Nobody would imagine giving or receiving massage over an open wound as it would be too painful for the patient and would cause a terrible mess! It is the most obvious contraindication and should be a matter of common sense. After a large wound has repaired there could be a residual problem due to scar tissue, which can be treated in a similar way to that described under Post-Operative Massage in Chapter 17.

Bone and joint injuries

Fractures
- Pain and tenderness around the injury site with any movement or weight-bearing
- Swelling and bruising in the injured area due to associated soft tissue damage
- Deformity and abnormal movement in fractured bone

Joint dislocation (subluxation)
- Severe dysfunction
- Severe pain
- Deformity

These conditions are not usually seen initially by a massage therapist, but if they are, then the history as well as the symptoms normally make them quite obvious. With fractures or dislocations of the wrist, fingers, ankle or toes, the symptoms may be less obvious, but if a fall or impact is involved it should always be considered first.

Massage in the acute stage of these conditions is obviously contraindicated as it would cause further damage. It would also cause the patient so much pain that he would not allow it to continue anyway.

Myositis ossificans

It is possible for a large haematoma that goes untreated for a long time to ossify and form into small pieces of bone material within the soft tissues. This is more likely to happen when a fracture has also been involved, as it could release osteoblasts into the tissues, which may be the catalyst for the calcification. Massage in this situation could cause the piece of bone to damage the surrounding soft tissues and so it is contraindicated.

Although this is a rare condition, it should be considered with patients who have had a long recovery from a serious fracture or other major trauma. Myositis ossificans usually shows up well on X-rays and so can easily be checked for, if in doubt.

Deep-vein thrombosis (DVT)

This is perhaps the most important contraindication that the massage therapist needs to be aware of, as failure to recognize it could have fatal consequences. A thrombosis (blood clot) can form in a vein and be dislodged, or a fragment (embolus) may break off, through the application of massage. As the veins get larger as they travel towards the heart, the clot will be able to pass unhindered along the system, through the chambers of the heart and into the pulmonary circulation. Here the vessels become smaller as they divide up into the lungs, and the clot will eventually get blocked as the vessels narrow, and will occlude an area of the lung. If it is a large clot, it will block the circulation to a major part of the lung (pulmonary embolism), or even to the whole lung, which could lead to death within minutes.

The factors that could lead to this condition are:

- Long periods of immobility or bed rest, which reduces circulation and can compress the veins
- Recent major surgery
- Varicose veins
- Heart disease
- Diabetes
- Contraceptive pill
- Impact trauma (which could cause damage inside the vein)

The veins usually affected are those in the calf and hamstring areas. Local pain and swelling are not always found, but this should only be true of patients who have had long periods of rest due to a serious illness or injury, in which case medical approval should always be sought first before treatment.

Although very rare, a DVT can occur in seemingly healthy people due to other predisposing factors. Acute pain and hard swelling may be felt when minimal pressure is applied, which in the first instance may give the appearance of an acute muscle strain. This does, however, feel quite different to the therapist who is used to feeling muscle injuries, as the area is much harder and has less secondary tension around it. There may also be some general swelling and discolouration to the distal part of the limb, due to restricted circulation. The patient may feel more pain and aching in the area when resting than would be expected if it were a muscle strain, and there would be no history to suggest such an injury either.

If a DVT is suspected, the patient should be referred to his doctor or hospital immediately.

Varicose veins

Varicose veins usually occur at the back of the leg. The valves within the veins, which prevent a back-flow in the circulation, break down and stop functioning. As the valve remains open, more blood and greater pressure is placed on the next valve back. The increased pressure affects the walls of the vein, which become stretched and eventually thicken and can become brittle.

Varicose veins can easily be seen as they look thick, dark blue, swollen and misshapen. But mild cases may be less noticeable, especially if the patient has already been lying on the treatment couch having massage for some time before the general condition of the leg is properly observed. And minor conditions may not cause discomfort, so the patient may be unaware of it or may simply forget to mention it.

In minor cases, light superficial stroking over the area should do no harm and may in fact ease the pressure off the vein and aid repair. Friction should not be applied, as this could further damage the walls of the blood vessels. In advanced cases, even superficial stroking should be avoided (there is the added risk of a DVT).

This contraindication relates only to the actual path of the vein itself; the tissues immediately adjacent to it can be treated. This will improve circulation away from the varicose vein and so relieve some of the pressure from it.

Infectious skin disease

Bacterial infection *Boils* are superficial abscesses that appear as a localized swelling on the skin, which eventually ruptures and discharges pus. *Folliculitis* is a condition when the hair follicles become inflamed and it appears as a rash of very small blisters. (This condition can be caused by deep massage if insufficient lubricant is used, particularly when treating men with hairy legs.) Massage can burst the blister(s), leaving the skin open to further infection (and can also create a rather unpleasant mess).

Lymphangitis Bacteria can invade the lymphatic system through open wounds, particularly if they have not been kept clean. The local area around the wound, which may itself be very minor, will appear red and swollen. A dark line can sometimes be seen running up the limb towards the lymph nodes, which may also be swollen and tender. Massage could spread the infection and the patient should seek medical treatment.

Fungal infection *Ringworm* and *athlete's foot* are the most common fungal infections and can affect warm, moist areas, such as between the toes, in the armpits or under the breast. The affected area may appear red with white flaky skin. Although massage does not worsen the problem, it can cause irritation and could be transmitted to the therapist's hands. For these reasons treatment is best avoided.

Viral infections Viral infections affecting the skin, such as *chicken pox* and *measles*, are common in children. In the early stages there may only be a mild skin rash, and it is possible that massage treatment may be requested for other reasons during this period. It is a contraindication because it can be transmitted to the therapist and should be considered if treating a child who has recently developed a rash.

Herpes Cold sores are the most common symptom of herpes and usually appear on the face and/or sacrum area. Before it erupts, the skin usually feels hyper-sensitive and tingling. Herpes is a virus that affects DNA and presently has no cure, and the cold sores will keep recurring from time to time. If present, any cold sores should be avoided because they will be very painful to the patient and there is a risk of transmission.

Other viral infections, such as *warts* and *verrucas*, should also be considered as contraindications, because the infection could be transmitted.

Melanoma (skin cancer)

Skin melanomas are becoming more common, probably because of the popularity of sun-tanning and travel to distant holiday locations, with sudden exposure to different climates. The diagnosis of these cancers is not the responsibility of the massage therapist, but it is important to be aware that they can occur in seemingly fit and healthy people who may seek massage for other reasons and do not know they could be developing this condition.

The common melanoma appears first as a change in pigmentation of the skin and looks like a large freckle. It should arouse suspicion if there is an increase in size or a change in shape, bleeding, itching or tingling. If given prompt medical treatment, this is an easily curable condition, but if left untreated it can have possibly fatal consequences.

Tumour

The massage therapist becomes used to examining the texture of the soft tissues very thoroughly and will find numerous small lumps within it. In most cases these can be explained as lesions relating to the musculoskeletal system. Some people also acquire small fatty nodules beneath the skin, which are soft, painless and move easily with the skin. These are harmless and can sometimes be broken down using friction techniques if they are bothering the patient.

Any other lumps are rare but could suggest a possible tumour. All lumps should be palpated carefully, and if they feel unusual and have no apparent history of a muscular skeletal cause, they should be referred to a medical practitioner. Massage, particularly friction, of a tumour could stimulate its development and help it spread to other areas and is therefore a definite contraindication.

Other cancers

People suffering from cancer should not receive massage as it may help spread its development through the body. A patient who is in remission may be able to have treatment but only under medical approval.

Bleeding disorders (haemophilia)

Haemophilia is a fairly rare hereditary disease, which prevents the ability of the blood to clot, and usually only affects males. There are several different types of the disease and each patient will suffer his own level of severity.

As the body has difficulty in stopping bleeding, anything that could cause trauma to the tissues, on any level, should be avoided. As deep massage can sometimes do this, haemophilia is a contraindication, depending on the severity of the disease. In mild cases it may be only deep friction that should be avoided, but in severe cases no massage can be considered safe. The patient's doctor will be able to advise on what is safe and possible.

Diabetes

Although diabetes is not actually a contraindication, there are factors that should be considered. The condition can affect the peripheral circulation, especially in the feet, causing the tissues to become more brittle and fragile. This can also affect the nerves and reduce the patient's sensitivity. Deep massage techniques can damage the brittle tissues and, with an impaired pain response, this may not be realized at the time.

The stimulating effect of massage on the circulation sometimes seems to have the same effect as exercise on the diabetic's blood sugar level. This need not be a problem, however, if the patient is warned of the possibility so that he is able to prepare his medication and/or diet accordingly.

4 The Working Posture

It is wrong to think of massage as something just done with the hands. The good therapist in fact uses his whole body, and the hands are just the sensitive 'machine heads' that come into contact with the patient.

Massage is a very physical therapy and as such can be considered almost a sport itself. As a treatment may take an hour, and a busy therapist may do perhaps eight or more treatments in a day, we are talking about a very aerobic type of activity. The muscles of the arms and hands are not particularly good aerobic muscles and very few arm exercises are carried out for more than about a minute at a time. Even a carpenter will not saw a piece of wood for long without stopping for a few seconds' rest. The large muscles of the legs and hips, however, are excellent aerobic muscles, which can function efficiently at a steady rate for many hours. In terms of power, too, the relatively small muscles of the arms would have to work at a maximal level to achieve any significant effect and would rapidly fatigue, but the larger muscles of the lower body can produce the same power by working at a much lower level. It therefore makes sense for the therapist to utilize the lower body as much as possible to generate the power behind all massage techniques.

But the muscles are not the only source of power available to the therapist. There is also body weight, which can be effortlessly added simply by leaning into the stroke. The key to good massage is to develop an efficient style, which achieves maximum power with minimum effort by combining the efficient use of muscle power and body weight.

Picture what happens when you push a heavy object: you do not stand very close and push just with the arms; instead you stand back, straighten the arms, lean your body weight forward, keep the back straight and then push through from your legs. This is virtually the same way that a massage therapist should perform long massage strokes up the body, with the arms and back straight and the movement coming from the legs and hips. This way very little effort is needed to achieve a powerful result. Body weight should be used properly by leaning into the stroke. At the end of the stroke it is necessary to push through the leading leg to extend the knee and return back to the starting position.

For transverse strokes across the body, the therapist should lean against the side of the couch and drop the body weight forward from the hips, keeping the arms and back straight, so that the weight is transmitted directly into the stroke. To return at the end of the stroke, the thighs can be pressed against the couch so that the therapist can straighten up by using the large hip extensor muscles. Very deep strokes can be made by gently pushing the stroke harder into the patient in order for the therapist to straighten up.

A common mistake often made by students is to lean very closely over the patient, with the elbows bent and the hands pointing inwards. This position makes massage very hard work and, apart from a close visual observation of the skin, has no benefits at all. It is extremely tempting for the student to concentrate on the actual hand techniques, but without good posture the hands may 'look' good but achieve very little.

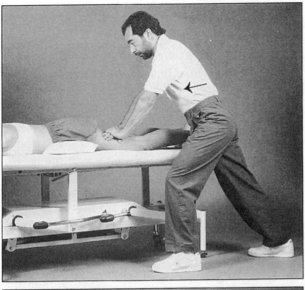

Keeping the arms, back and back leg straight, the therapist can apply long strokes by shifting his body weight forward onto the front leg and allowing the front knee to flex.

As there is an infinite variety of massage strokes, it is impossible to describe all the working postures. But at all times the therapist should focus on keeping a well-balanced stance, with the knees slightly bent and the hips square and facing the direction of the stroke. Rather than twisting the body to work in different directions, the feet should keep moving so that the hips remain squarely behind the stroke. The upper body should maintain a steady, repetitive rhythm and it is the legs and feet that move to change the direction of the stroke and the area being treated. Not only does this achieve excellent results, but it also helps to keep the therapist fit.

It is important for the therapist to try and keep his upper back straight at all times and not allow it to bend as he works over the couch, as this can eventually cause chronic aching in the mid-thoracic area (a common complaint among busy therapists). In an effort to concentrate treatment effectively on specific areas such as the neck, however, it is

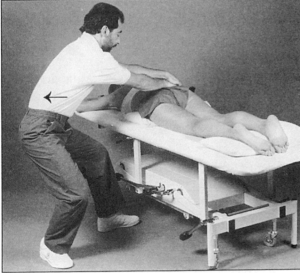

Here the stroke is pulled back across the body. The therapist pushes through the front (left) leg and creates the movement by flexing the back (right) knee.

almost impossible to avoid this. In these situations the therapist can kneel with one knee on the couch. This shifts the body weight forward so that the centre of gravity is much closer to the area being treated, and enables work to continue with a straight back. Some therapists now work using a very low couch so that they can adopt this position most of the time, and this can be helpful in preventing back problems.

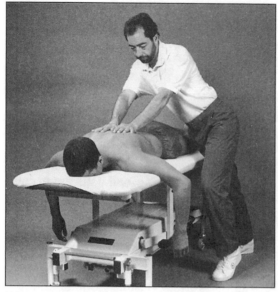

When working up the back it is necessary to lean across the couch to get the body weight central above the patient.

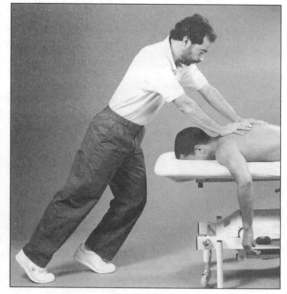

Deep stroking using considerable weight and force through the heel of the leading hand (push through the other hand to return).

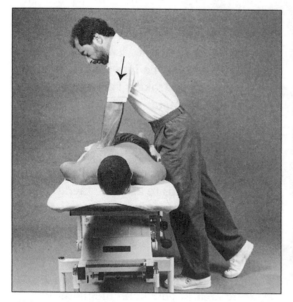

With a straight back and arms, deep transverse strokes can be applied by simply dropping the body weight down onto the patient.

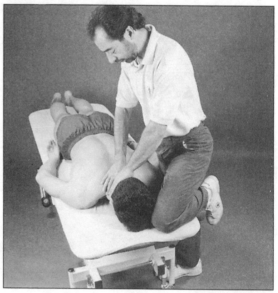

Placing one knee on the couch moves the centre of gravity much closer to the patient, so that the therapist does not have to lean over so much when concentrating on a central area like the neck.

A good working posture achieves far more than just power and efficiency, it also greatly enhances the quality of touch and feel. As the whole body is involved in the stroke, any changes in the texture or tension of the tissues can be felt through the senses in the therapist's whole body, not just the hands and arms.

Kneeling positions are
sometimes useful. Deep
strokes can be applied
through straight arms by
moving the body forward
onto the front leg.

There are other benefits too, which can be explained in terms of the martial art of Taiqi. Those familiar with this art will see close similarities with the working postures described here for massage. By being well 'centred' and 'grounded', the Qi energy (or life force) flows freely through the therapist's body and into the patient. Quite simply, the therapeutic quality of touch becomes much greater by adding this vital form of energy.

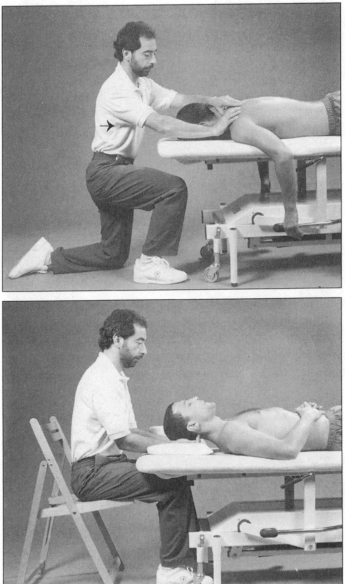

Energy is an important factor in the treatment process. Therapists sometimes find that after treating a particular patient they feel drained and exhausted even though it may not have been especially hard work. This is probably because the patient had a very low level of Qi energy and they literally drained it from the therapist. A good working posture that allows a free flow of Qi energy will not only give the patient what he needs, but will also not drain energy from the therapist.

The importance of a good working posture for the therapist cannot be emphasized strongly enough, because without it massage is hard work and not very effective. With it, massage becomes effortless, instinctive and extremely powerful.

Floor-work

Massage does not need to be done on a treatment couch and this gives the therapist the freedom to work almost anywhere (even up a mountain!). When treating a patient on the floor the therapist

Sitting on a chair
can be useful when
concentrating on an area
like the neck.

needs to get into a comfortable position, but this does not mean sitting astride the patient.

To work up the back, the therapist should place one knee to the side of the patient's waist and his other foot just below the armpit on the other side of the patient's body. In this position long strokes can be applied by leaning down through the arms onto the patient and lunging

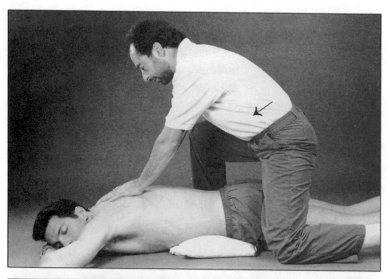

Strokes can be applied by moving the body forward and flexing the front knee.

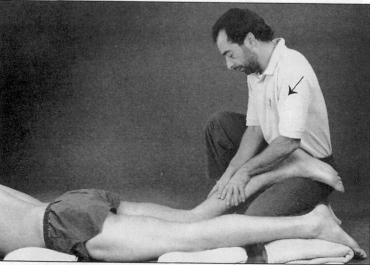

Supporting the lower leg on the thigh of the therapist's kneeling leg, which takes away the need to bend down to treat the area. Strokes are applied along the muscle by moving the body forward and down.

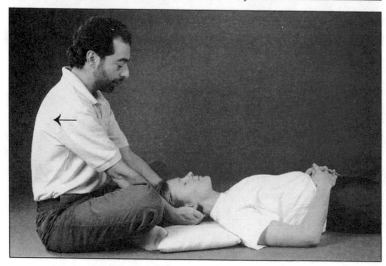

Sitting cross-legged at the patient's head to work the muscles of the neck. Strokes are applied by leaning back (a very peaceful position).

forward from the hips, the weight being transferred from the back knee onto the front foot.

This is an excellent position to work in as the therapist's body is centred directly over the patient and almost the full body weight can be used. Some therapists who are physically small may find that working on the floor is actually preferable for this reason. Occasionally a therapist may even climb onto the couch to use this position to get more weight behind a technique.

Working from the side, the therapist can kneel very close to the patient and place his hands on the body. With his arms straight, the therapist can rise up from his knees and lean down onto the patient to apply deep transverse techniques (see example on p. 51).

5 Palpation

Identifying changes in texture, tension or actual damage in the soft tissues is of course a very important part of massage. Sometimes the affected areas are fairly large and can easily be felt by the patients themselves without the need for any specially developed skill. But the professional therapist needs to assess the tissues on a microscopic level to be able to identify the very specific tissues that may be at the root of the problem. Sometimes it could be just a few fibres no thicker than a human hair that are damaged and causing the trouble, and it requires a high level of palpatory skill to identify these. As with any human skill, this can be developed through practice and also by using some specific exercises.

It is necessary to identify very localized areas that feel irregular or different, compared to the adjacent tissues. The patient's pain perception is important in helping in this identification process. As well as asking for verbal feedback, there are non-verbal clues such as facial expression, clenching the fist or curling the toes. While applying deep palpation through one hand, the therapist's other hand should be in gentle contact with the patient. In this way it is often possible to sense a pain response and it also reassures the patient that the intention is not just one of brutality.

Pain alone does not necessarily mean that there is a problem, as there are trigger-points in the body that are naturally a little painful when deeply palpated. And there are certain tissues, such as the iliotibial band, which naturally need a fairly high degree of tension for normal function, and this can feel painful when pressed deeply. If the tissues feel normal to the therapist but cause pain when palpated, compare them with the other side of the body. If there is a difference, then there may be a problem to treat; if they feel the same, this can reassure the patient that there is no problem and that the feeling is normal.

There is no benefit in just applying deep passive pressure in a small area and then releasing it, because this only shows what those particular tissues feel like and gives no information about how they compare with the surrounding tissues. Instead, it is necessary to press into the tissues and then, maintaining this pressure, to use the plasticity of the skin and subcutaneous layers to glide in all directions throughout the area to feel any textural changes.

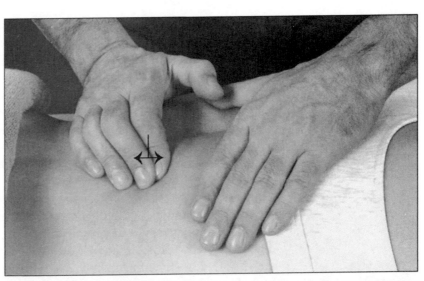

The palpating tip of the forefinger is being supported by the other fingers. Passive pressure is applied into the tissues, and then gliding movements are made to identify any textural changes.

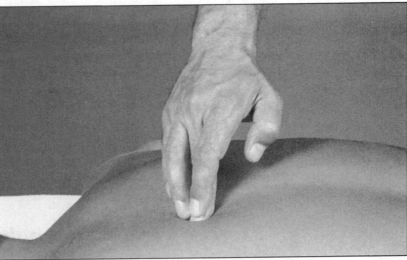

The palpating middle fingertip is strengthened and supported by the other fingers.

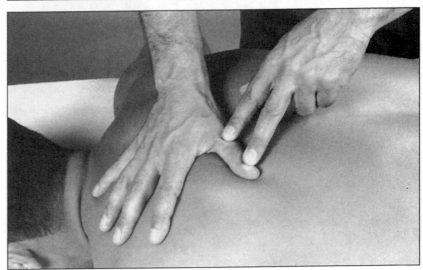

The joints of the palpating thumb should be protected. Although this picture shows this being done with the fingers of the other hand, more power can be applied using the heel of the palm instead, but in this position the thumb cannot be seen.

Damage can occur at any level, and although most problems tend to be found on a deep level, this is not always the case. One mistake sometimes made is to explore deeper and deeper into the tissues in an effort to find the problem, only to miss it because it is located more superficially. It is therefore necessary to vary the degree of pressure used from fairly light to very deep to assess all the different tissue layers.

As well as the soft tissues, it is necessary to feel the surfaces of the bony structures where fibrosis or scar tissue may also occur (for example, the medial border of the tibia). When palpating around a joint it is good to move it into different positions, as this gives access to different surfaces of the bones and soft tissues.

Although the tips of the fingers or thumb are usually used for palpation, to apply deeper pressure or to prevent injury to the therapist's digits, the elbow can be used instead to great effect (the knee and foot are also used by some therapists). When first using the elbow there will probably be little diagnostic sensitivity, but with practice it can become just as sensitive as a fingertip.

The thumb is perhaps the most common tool used for applying very deep pressure, and without good technique therapists often suffer from chronic inflammation in the joints. It is vital to keep the thumb fairly relaxed and to use it as a passive tool, with the power coming from the other hand bearing down on it. Not only does this protect the thumb joints from compression force but, being relaxed, the thumb is also more sensitive.

Therapists with hyper-flexibility in the wrist and fingers must ensure that heavy pressure is applied only when the joints are held in a fairly straight position, otherwise they may suffer injury.

Exercises to develop palpatory skill

Put some small pieces of different materials, such as wood, plastic, stone and metal, in your pocket. Keep taking a piece between your fingers and feeling its shape, texture and temperature. Use smaller and smaller pieces as your skill increases. Eventually it is possible to actually sense the shape of a piece of grit, or a grain of salt or sand.

Place some coins of different sizes and thicknesses between different pages of a magazine. Try to feel and identify the coins and their depth within the magazine.

Masseur's party game

Get someone to take a single hair from the head, put it on a table and cover it with a sheet of newspaper (without you seeing). Then try to feel where the hair is. Try this again using two sheets of newspaper, and so on.

6 General Massage Techniques

As with any sector of the population, massage therapists come in many different shapes and sizes, with differing strengths, weaknesses and flexibility. The hands are a good example of how different people can be. Comparing the degree of extension possible at the wrist, finger and thumb joints shows enormous differences, and therapists need to develop their own unique style, which takes account of this. Although great flexibility may mean that the hands are able to perform more versatile massage strokes, there are potential dangers. Repetitive pressure through hyper-extended joints can eventually cause damage to the tendons of the wrist flexors and inflammation of finger and thumb joints.

For students who may be practising only a few hours a week, these problems may not be immediately apparent, and so they may develop techniques and habits that prove to be harmful in the future. Many talented therapists have had their careers shortened due to chronic hand injuries and so this must be a primary consideration. Care should always be taken to protect the joints by not having them hyper-extended when applying techniques requiring heavy pressure, such as deep stroking and friction. Ideally in these situations, the bones of the arm, wrist and fingers should be fixed in an almost straight line so that the force is direct and there is minimal stress on the joint structures.

Stroking (effleurage)

This is the principal diagnostic and treatment technique used in massage and can be performed in an infinite variety of ways. The basic variables of application are:

- Pressure: superficial or deep
- Direction: longitudinal or transverse (to muscle fibres)

Longitudinal – superficial This technique is used in a general way at the start of treatment to spread the oil and give initial warmth and comfort. The strokes should be performed with the palms of both hands covering a large area. More pressure is applied with a long, upward stroke towards the heart (when treating a limb) and lighter pressure on the return stroke. *The pressure stroke must always be applied* up *a limb* (see General Circulation in Chapter 2).

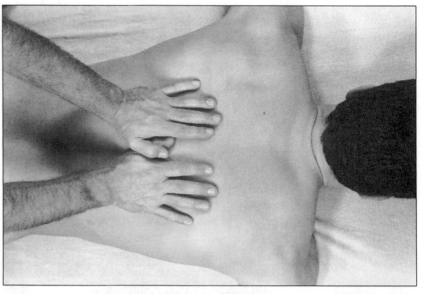

Using the palms and fingers of both hands to stroke up the erector spinae muscles.

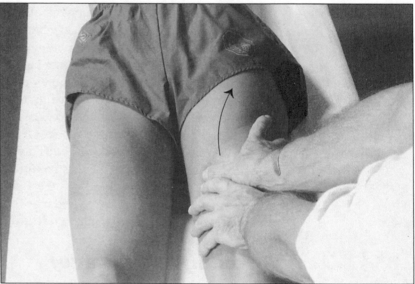

Using the palms and fingers of both hands to stroke up the quadriceps.

The hands stay in contact with the skin at all times. At the end of the pressure stroke it is more pleasant to make a rounded, sweeping movement than a sudden stop and change direction. Pressure should be focused through the heel of the palms rather than in the fingers, as this provides a more efficient transfer of power from the arms. The fingers should be relaxed so that the hands mould themselves smoothly over the contours of the area being treated. The actual movement behind the stroke comes through the whole body, from the legs, and the arms themselves should actually move very little (see Chapter 4).

These strokes should run the full length of the muscles from attachment to attachment and should be slow enough to allow good observa-

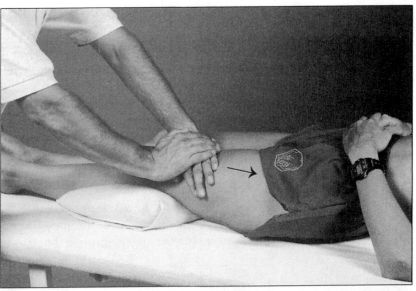

A deeper stroke can be applied by placing one hand on top of the other.

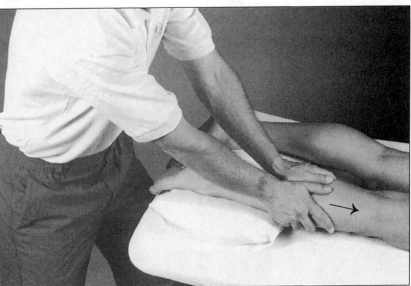

Using the palms and fingers of both hands to stroke up the calf muscles.

tion of how the tissues feel. By doing this over a large area it should be possible for the therapist to detect general areas that feel harder or tighter than adjacent areas.

To apply deeper strokes it is not necessary to use more force, just a smaller area of contact. By putting one hand on top of the other with the same effort, the therapist will achieve a deeper and more focused stroke. The area of contact can be further reduced by using just the pad on the outside edge of the palm (between the little finger and wrist) or the thenar eminence (the pad between the thumb and wrist).

These strokes should be repeated many times, proceeding systematically across the specific part of the body but concentrating more on any areas that feel harder or tighter.

The primary effect of these effleurage strokes is to pump the circulation and to identify general areas of tension. These strokes create the general 'back-cloth' to the whole massage treatment and should be returned to constantly in between other techniques. Deeper work may loosen adhered fibres and break down scar tissue but will cause discomfort, while these superficial strokes will flush the circulation through the area, clearing away any particles loosened by deeper techniques and relaxing the tissues again.

Transverse – superficial

The hands are used in exactly the same ways as above, but strokes are applied across the direction of the muscle fibres.

When treating the legs, transverse strokes can also be applied by grasping around the belly of the muscle and using the thumb as an anchor, drawing the fingers through the tissues towards the thumb. This

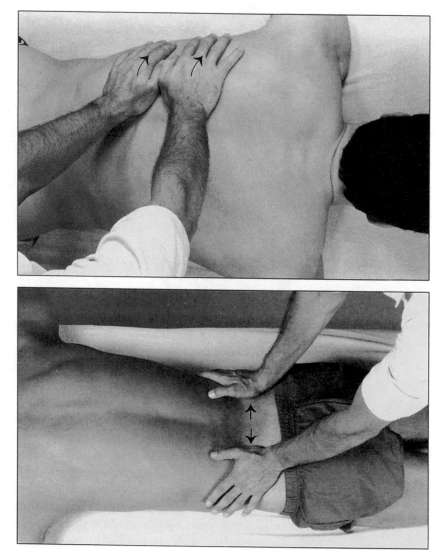

A transverse stroke with the heels of both palms, from the spine and across the erector spinae and latissimus dorsi muscles.

Bilateral transverse stroking of the hips and lower back.

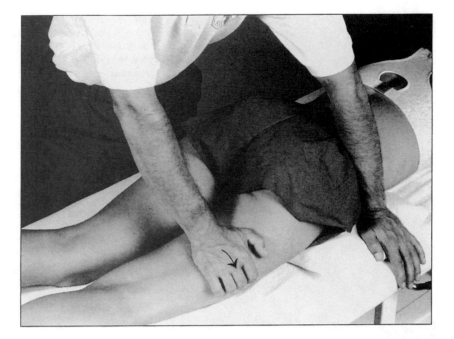

Transverse stroking with the heel of the palm drawing towards the fingers.

can also be done the other way, with the thumb being drawn towards the fingers (stopping before pinching the skin).

The effect of transverse stokes on the circulation is not as strong as longitudinal strokes, but they are very good diagnostically. Tension in the soft tissues tends to build up in bands running lengthwise through the muscle. As the stroke crosses the muscle, these bands can be felt more easily as they do not pass as smoothly under the hand. Transverse strokes also help to loosen and separate individual muscles and compartments, which may be binding together.

Longitudinal and transverse – deep

Progressively smaller contact points can be used to move deeper into the tissues. For this the pad or tip of the thumb, fingers or even the elbow can be used. As these strokes are deep they will stretch the tissues, so they should become shorter (down to just a few inches/centimetres) the deeper they go, to prevent local over-stretching.

Great care must be taken not to cause excessive pain and also to protect the finger or thumb of the therapist. The working digit should be used as a passive tool, with the power coming from the other hand, which presses on it as close to the tip as possible. Because the digit in contact with the client is relaxed, it is much more sensitive and better able to feel and work the tissues.

These deep stroking techniques are the most effective way to identify deep lesions and should be performed slowly to enable good observation. Where lesions are located, a combination of longitudinal and transverse stokes can be used. *Transverse* strokes will break the bonds (adhesions) between the fibres and *longitudinal* strokes will stretch and realign them. They also stimulate the local circulation.

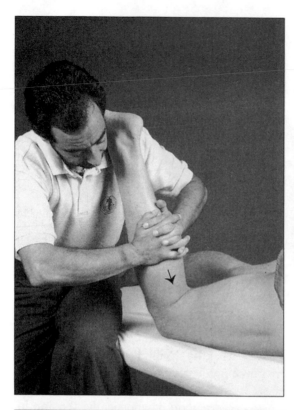

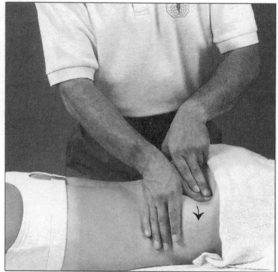

Left: The heels of both hands can squeeze the muscles in a vice-like action, and the stroke is made downwards towards the knee. The lower leg is relaxed in an elevated position by resting the patient's foot on the therapist's shoulder.

Below: Deep stroking with the thumb, supported by the fingers of the other hand.

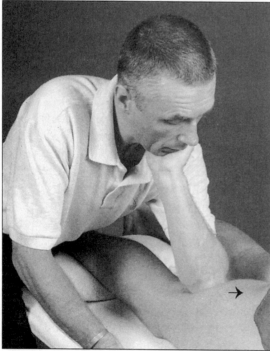

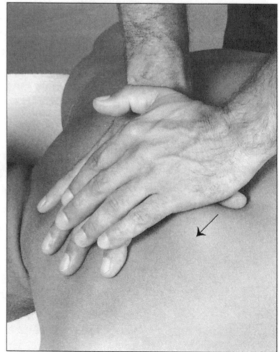

Deep stroking can be applied very slowly using an elbow. Even more pressure can be applied by resting the weight of the head on the hand.

Deep stroking, keeping the thumb relaxed so that it acts like a passive tool, while the power behind the stroke comes through the heel of the overlying hand.

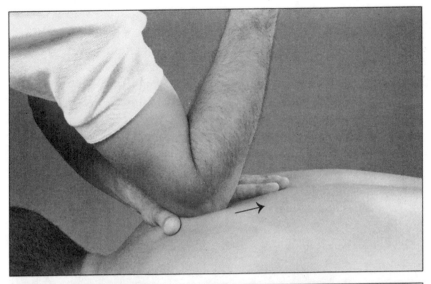

Deep stroking with the tip of the elbow. The other hand is used to create a pocket around the elbow to guide and control the stroke.

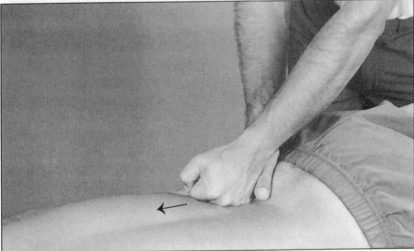

With the elbow and wrist held straight, the fist can be used to apply deep strokes. The other hand can be used to guide the stroke.

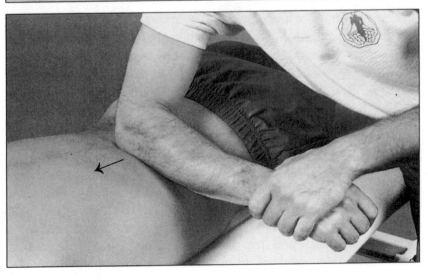

Deep stroking with the ulnar border of the forearm. The other hand can be used to vary the angle of the forearm according to the contours of the body, and also for adjusting the pressure.

Cam and spindle

This is a deep stroking technique in which the therapist uses the thumb of one hand as a 'cam' or pivot, with the other hand forming a loose fist around it to act as a 'spindle'. The 'cam' hand makes a gliding stroke up the limb while the knuckles of the 'spindle' hand stroke deeply into the muscle while rotating round the thumb. To work even deeper on specific bands of tension the therapist can use three, two or just one finger as the spindle around the thumb.

The 'cam and spindle' technique: while one hand guides the stroke and the thumb provides the spindle, the fist of the other hand twists round the thumb to stroke very deeply into the muscle.

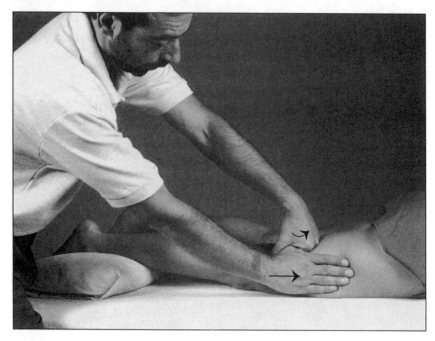

Kneading (petrissage)

This is performed with both hands working together in a smooth, rhythmical way. Each hand in turn is opened fully to grasp across the muscle, then squeezes and lifts the tissues. As one hand releases its grip, the other takes up a grip adjacent to it, very much like kneading dough. A steady rhythm should be maintained with the two hands, and the technique should slowly travel up and down the specific part of the body. This is particularly easy on areas like the legs and top of the shoulders, but with practice it can also become a satisfying technique to apply to all areas. As skill develops, it becomes possible to isolate and treat quite small muscles using the tips of the thumb and fingers.

This technique stimulates the circulation, generally loosens and softens the tissues, and has a great warming effect. If, however, the tissues are excessively tense through minor injury or fatigue, petrissage may feel unpleasant and irritating. If this is the case, more superficial stroking should be used first before attempting to knead again.

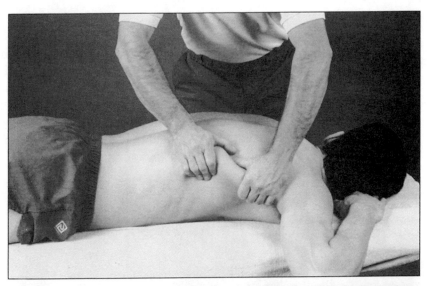

Kneading (petrissage) on the latissimus dorsi muscle.

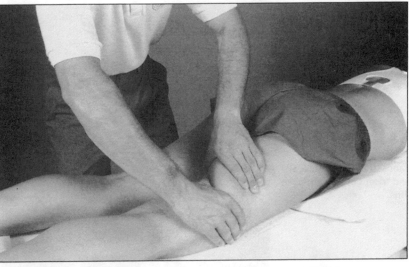

Kneading (petrissage) on the hamstring muscles.

Kneading (petrissage) the adductor muscles. (The therapist has one knee on the couch and is supporting the patient's leg on his thigh.)

Squeezing

Because of the system of non-return valves in the blood vessels, a squeezing action has a pumping effect on the circulation.

When squeezing the tissues it is important not to dig in with the fingertips. The movement should take place between the thumb and thenar eminence and all of the fingers (held straight rather than hooked). This technique has the advantage of being just as effective when applied through clothing.

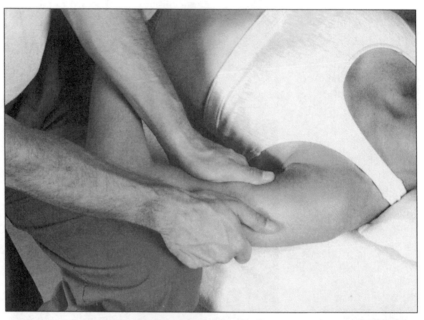

Squeezing with both hands, treating the biceps and triceps at the same time.

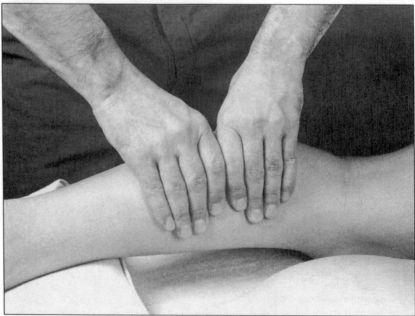

Squeezing the calf muscles between the fingers and thumbs of both hands.

Friction

This is the deepest technique used in massage and is targeted at specific areas of soft tissue damage, such as scar tissue and adhesions. The digit or elbow is used in a similar way as with deep effleurage, but even greater pressure is applied. It is first applied passively until sufficient depth has been reached, and any lesions can then be located and treated by using a friction, rotation or short rocking movement while maintaining the same deep pressure. The depth of the friction can

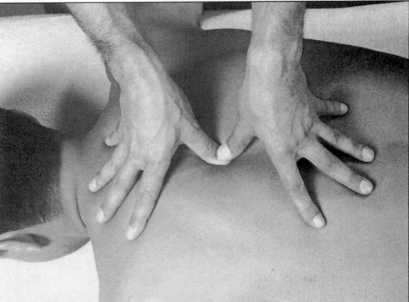

Friction with one thumb on top of the other. The fingers are splayed out for support and control.

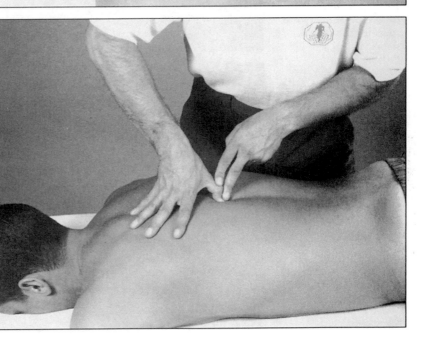

Friction with the tip of the thumb strengthened by the fingers of the other hand.

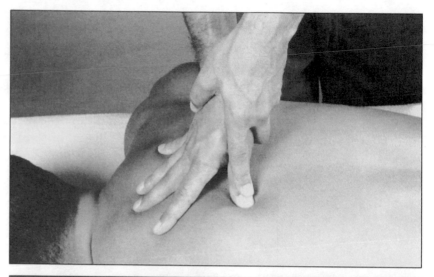

Friction with the thumb, supported by the other fingers and strengthened by the other hand.

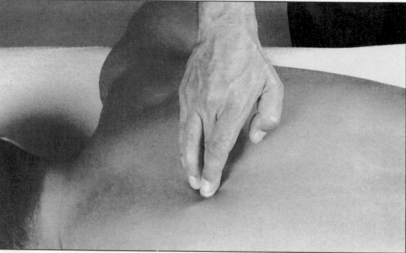

Friction with the fingertip, supported by the other fingers.

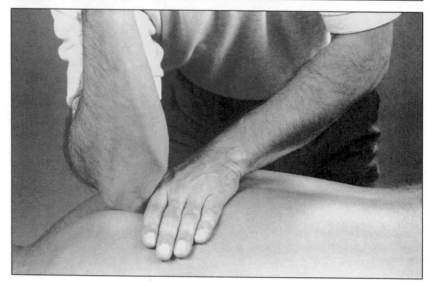

Friction with the tip of the elbow. The other hand is used to control the movement.

change with the angle between the working digit and the surface of the skin. Applying friction directly into the tissues at 90 degrees penetrates the most deeply, but care must be taken not to bruise the tissues by squashing them against bone.

Great sensitivity is required to use as much pressure as possible, but staying just within pain tolerance. Friction is a very powerful technique, which can damage the tissues if used too forcefully. It should never be applied to acute conditions, and only with caution in the early recovery stage.

Even with correct use, friction is a painful technique that may sometimes cause bruising, and it is worth advising the patient of this at the time.

When working on areas of scar tissue, friction should be applied for only short periods of time (about one minute), otherwise the tissues may become irritated and a local reflex muscle contraction may occur. The same area can be returned to again for further friction treatment several times during a single session, and frequently a noticeable change in the tissues appears to take place during those short rest periods in between.

When treating large, knotted areas of compacted fibrous tissue, the fingers of the skilled therapist can feel its shape. By concentrating friction into the narrow parts and indentations, it may be possible to break it into smaller and looser lumps. The blood will then be able to flow more freely through the area, stimulating the healing process and continuing the breakdown process naturally.

Friction is an excellent diagnostic technique, which has several therapeutic effects. As well as breaking down scar tissue and adhesions, it loosens and re-aligns tangled fibres and stimulates local circulation. It is used not only on specific target areas within the larger soft tissue areas, but also generally around joints to stimulate circulation and release fibrous adhesions there, too.

Friction is also used in neuromuscular techniques, where it is often applied for much longer periods. For example, when stimulating golgi tendon organs (at the tendon insertions) Dr James Cyriax advocated friction for up to 15 minutes, although many therapists and patients may find this excessive.

Deep friction often requires the heaviest pressure of all the massage techniques and, as it is usually applied through a single digit, the greatest care must be taken to protect the joints of that digit. Some therapists use a stick or similar device to apply deep friction, but with good technique this should rarely be necessary. It is better to develop good elbow techniques so that you do not have to rely on your fingers or thumb (or any device) and risk joint problems.

Areas that have been treated with deep friction should be stretched afterwards, either with deep and superficial longitudinal strokes and/or passive and functional stretches.

Rocking and shaking

These techniques are commonly used in massage and appeal to the senses on perhaps a more primary level, like rocking a baby.

Rocking can be done with the hands applying firm but gentle pressure over a whole part of the body (leg or back usually). The hands rock the body, working either together or in opposite directions to create

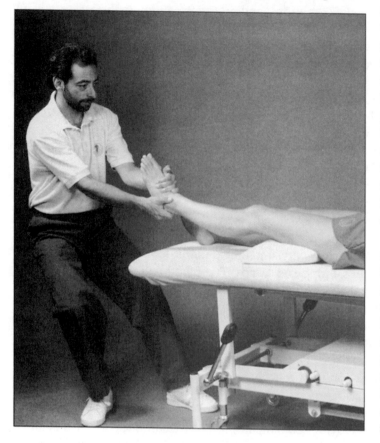

a smooth, wave-like motion through the whole area. This is an excellent way of starting and finishing the treatment of an area, particularly when done through a towel. It is sometimes performed during treatment if the client has generally tightened up because of discomfort during deep massage. Rocking can even be used at the same time as deep friction to encourage relaxation.

Shaking can be carried out on a whole limb by grasping firmly around the ankle or wrist, raising the limb and applying a mild traction (pull). The whole limb can be shaken quite vigorously, usually in the horizontal plane through a fairly short range. This can have an excellent effect on overall relaxation or stimulation, depending on speed, and can loosen the joints.

Percussion (tapotement)

Percussion techniques are made with alternate hands striking the skin in very rapid succession. Although this may look rather violent, it is in fact very light and stimulating. The rapid action comes from the elbow, with the wrist remaining fairly loose, and the hands withdraw as soon as they strike the surface of the skin.

Cupping (clapping) is probably the most common form of percussion. The hands are formed into a shallow cup shape, so that a pocket of air is trapped against the skin as the hand strikes. This creates a deep but soft percussion effect and should make a hollow sound, not a slapping sound.

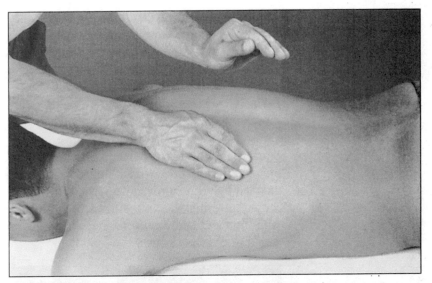

Percussion: cupping.

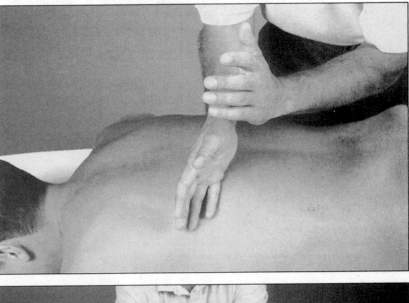

Percussion: hacking.

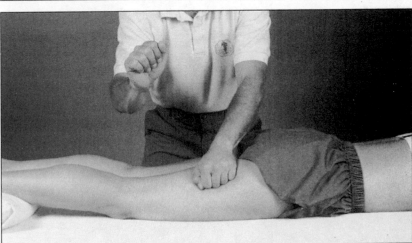

Percussion: beating.

Hacking is performed with the ulnar (outside) border of the hand. The wrists must be held loosely to prevent a heavy chopping action. A more vibrating effect can be achieved by striking the surface with loosely held fingers.

Beating is carried out by striking lightly with the palmar surface of a loosely held fist.

Shearing is not strictly a percussion technique but it also involves rapid movement and produces a similar effect. The belly of the muscle is grasped by both hands close together. One hand then makes a sudden thrust, pushing the tissues away, while the other pulls them back. Although sudden, the thrust should not be forced beyond the natural resistance in the tissues.

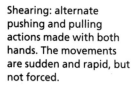

Shearing: alternate pushing and pulling actions made with both hands. The movements are sudden and rapid, but not forced.

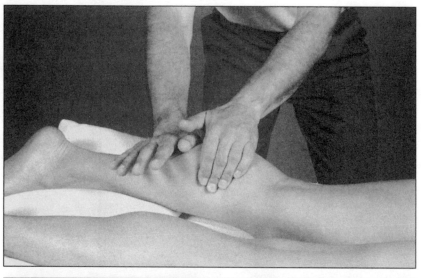

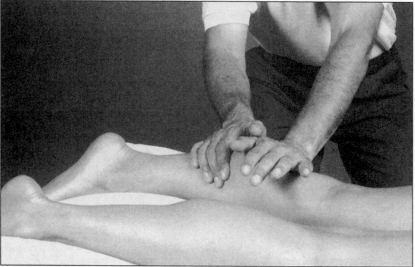

These percussion techniques can be highly stimulating and are often not considered appropriate because relaxation is felt to be more important. But they can be used to help wake a patient up before he leaves, and in competitive sporting situations such stimulation can be a very important pre-event technique. It is also helpful with some nerve conditions such as multiple sclerosis, and can help nerve stimulation and muscle contraction following a period of immobilization.

Although percussion is always considered a stimulating technique, when applied slowly with fairly heavy contact it can be highly relaxing. Sometimes a muscle that is in spasm can be released in this way.

Working through clothing

Massage involves the manual treatment of the soft tissues using whatever practical means. The use of oils and making direct contact with the patient's skin simply represent the conventional way in which it is performed. Equally effective treatment can be done through clothing without using oil, so the therapist should not consider himself tied to equipment but able to work anywhere. One of my own hobbies has been climbing in the Himalayas and I have occasionally needed to give treatment in very extreme situations. Nobody would take their clothes off in sub-zero temperatures, or attempt to carry a massage couch up a glacier, but this in no way restricted the use of massage (see Floor-work in Chapter 4).

The only massage technique that cannot be applied through clothes is long stroking – everything else adapts very easily. Squeezing and kneading techniques will stimulate blood-flow and have a warming and

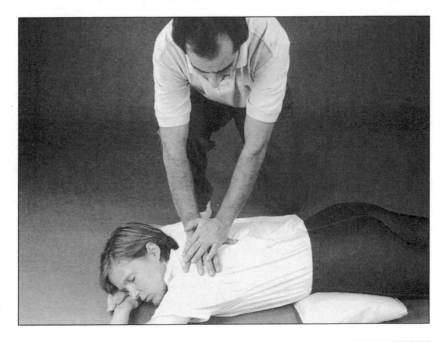

Deep pressure with short gliding movements applied through clothing to the thoracic area of the back.

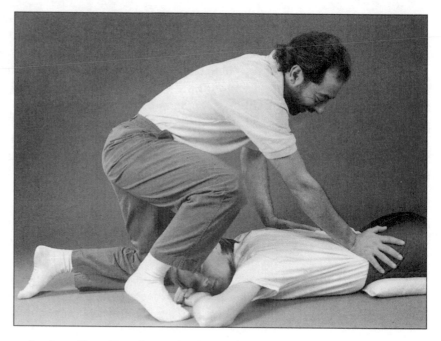

Deep pressure and short strokes through clothing, to the lower back and hip.

softening effect. To palpate the tissues it is necessary to apply deep pressure and then glide along the deeper layers to feel any areas of damage. Clothing can provide a good grip with the skin and actually make this easier to do. Even in a conventional treatment, using oil, it is sometimes better to work through a towel when applying very deep techniques, as this provides better grip and control.

Rhythm and speed

Developing a good rhythm is an important part of massage. It not only creates a more flowing technique, but also enables the patient to anticipate the stroke and relax into it better.

Speed is one of the key variables in creating the desired overall effect of massage. Generally a slow pace is more relaxing and a fast pace more stimulating. The speed can even be varied during a treatment to suit particular requirements. For example, a patient who has to return to work after treatment can have deep, relaxing massage at the beginning and fast, stimulating massage to wake him up at the end.

When applying deep massage techniques it is important to work slowly. Not only does this allow good observation on a very detailed level, but also enables the patient to cope better with the technique. A fast, deep stroke can cause a sudden sharp pain when it hits a lesion, and this can result in local or general reflex muscle contraction, which prevents good treatment. By working slowly, the patient has time to prepare and relax into the stroke or friction and to suppress reflex activity. This also enables a neuromuscular reaction to take place (see Chapter 14).

Massage treatment

'The whole is greater than the sum of its parts.'

A treatment is more than a collection of different techniques; it is the combination of these techniques that adds a new dimension. Any constant stroke applied for a long period will become irritating, so it is necessary to keep changing them. Even using a variety of strokes on a small general area, like a hip or a thigh, may cause irritation after a few minutes of constant attention. But to complicate matters, it is also important not to change technique or move to another area too quickly, because the client needs time to relax into the technique before it can have any real effect.

Another reason to keep changing strokes is because tension reduces in stages. It often feels as though little improvement is taking place while the tissues are actually being treated, but when they are returned to a few minutes later a noticeable relaxation does appear to have occurred. It is as if the nervous system adapts to the change in tissue condition after the 'assault' of the treatment has finished. So each time that an area is returned to for concentrated attention, it should be possible to work on a deeper level. And as the tension releases, the deeper tissues become easier to assess. Sometimes an area has to be returned to many times, and it is only at the end that there is sufficient relaxation for the therapist actually to feel a tiny lesion that may be causing the problem.

There is no simple way of explaining how to do this as it is purely a matter of instinct and experience. It is necessary to sense the reaction in the tissues being treated as well as in the patient as a whole, and to make a change just before these reactions become negative. This may sound vague and unscientific, but in this natural therapy the key to good results will always involve a degree of instinct.

General procedure (limbs)

When treating a limb there is a basic procedure that must be followed. The proximal part (thigh or upper arm) should receive stroking massage techniques before any treatment is given to the distal part. This is to clear the lymph vessels and stimulate circulation so that fluids from the distal part can escape more freely when it is treated. When concentrating on a problem in the distal part, the proximal part should be returned to every few minutes, with long, stroking techniques, to maintain a good through-flow of fluids.

Routine

There is *no* standard routine for massage, as it should depend entirely on the individual situation. The priority must always be to treat the pain first, but time must always be found also to treat adjacent areas, as part of the problem may be found there. It is also important to treat the same area on the other side of the body for comparative purposes.

The part of the body that the therapist decides is the focus of the treatment is usually treated first. This enables more time to be spent there and gives an opportunity to return to it several times during the session. For example, with a hamstring injury, treatment can start with an initial assessment and superficial techniques on the injured area. Then the other leg can be treated, before returning to the injury for deeper treatment. Next the back and hip can be treated, before returning to the injury for a third time.

Sometimes the therapist may want to start by working on another area first to help the patient relax generally, and then proceed to work on the injury area.

Student's note: Giving massage is like being a blind artist; you never know just what your work feels like. Practise on a friend who will give honest feedback. Experiment with different ways of doing things and ask what feels best. Try this on different people and you will probably get different answers. No two people will respond in quite the same way. That is why every massage should be unique.

7 General Abdomen Massage

The abdomen is dealt with separately as it involves different considerations from the rest of the body. Massage should *not* be carried out during pregnancy, as the pressure could disturb the foetus. Although it is not contraindicated during normal menstruation, women often find it unpleasant at this time, although sometimes it can prove to be very helpful.

The abdomen is often not included in a general massage treatment, especially when other musculoskeletal problems are a priority. This is usually due to limited time, or because the patient may not expect or request it. But it has many benefits and should be used whenever possible. As well as the effect it can have locally, abdomen massage can greatly enhance overall relaxation. The abdomen is a vulnerable part of the body, which we instinctively protect from external forces. Excessive tension often occurs here and goes unnoticed, not just for direct physical reasons but also in response to emotional stress. To accept the physical application of massage, the patient has to overcome the reflex to tense the muscles more and actually relax them instead. The effect of this can be quite profound and can lead to a more long-term improvement in general relaxation and well-being.

If the muscles are tight, increased abdominal pressure resists the downward pull of the diaphragm, which can restrict inhalation. If they are weak, they are less able to increase abdominal pressure and assist forced exhalation. By treating the abdomen it is therefore possible to improve respiration.

Massage can also aid digestion and help minor abdominal problems. It can do this by relaxing and toning the surrounding muscles, stimulating the circulation of blood and intestinal fluids, and releasing fibrous adhesions around organs and other tissues (see Chapter 17).

General treatment

To treat the abdomen the patient should be in a supine position, with the hips and knees considerably flexed and the feet flat on the couch. The head, neck and upper back should also be raised and comfortably supported. This shortens and helps relax the muscles, making it possible to treat the tissues properly.

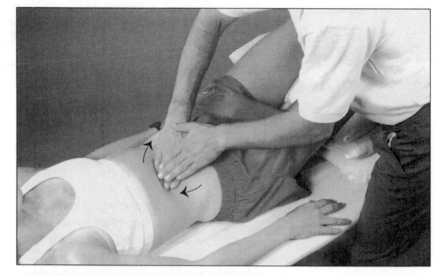

Superficial stroking in a clockwise direction using the pads of the fingers supported by the other hand.

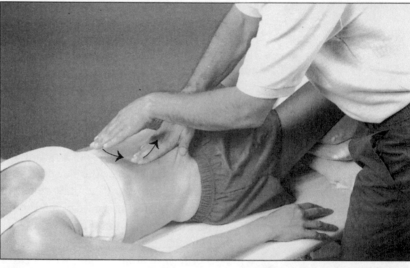

Stroking with alternate hands from the outer borders of the abdomen, travelling clockwise, in towards the umbilicus.

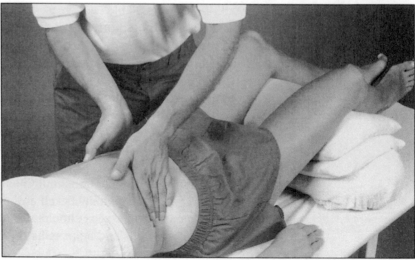

Deep transverse strokes (bilateral) can be applied from the back all the way to the umbilicus, lifting the tissues along the way.

The most important feature of massage treatment is the direction of the long strokes, which *must* go in a *clockwise* direction to follow the large intestines (colon). Starting from the right inguinal area, just above the iliac crest, strokes should travel up along the ascending colon to the bottom right rib (and slightly beneath it if possible). Then along the transverse colon to the left rib (and under it if possible), before going down the descending colon to the left inguinal area. To work in the opposite direction would cause a potentially harmful back-flow of substances into the small intestines.

Deep kneading (petrissage) is an excellent technique for treating the abdominal area deeply.

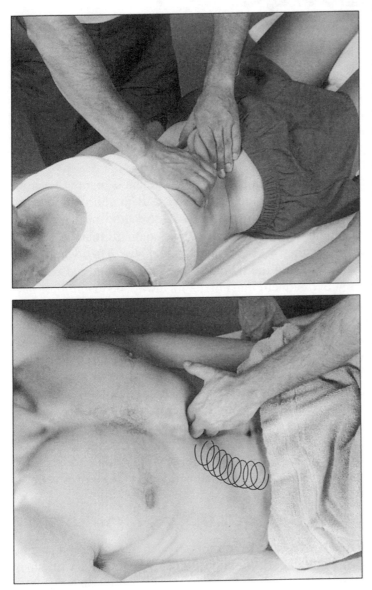

The pressure of the stroke should be reduced as it passes across the solar plexus area, just below the base of the sternum (xiphoid cartilage). At the end of the stroke (left inguinal area) pressure should be removed so that the hands pass lightly across the bladder area to begin the next stroke on the right side again. These strokes should start off gently but, as the patient relaxes, providing there is no pain, the pressure can be increased very considerably. Once softened with stroking, deep kneading works very well.

Friction can also be applied gently along the colon using the back of the knuckles and making small rotational movements at the wrist.

Deep friction techniques are difficult if the muscles are too relaxed, because the pressure simply pushes the muscle into the soft underlying viscera. This also makes it difficult to identify whether any discomfort is coming from the muscle or an underlying organ. Pain from a soft tissue injury will increase if the muscle contracts while being palpated, by the patient flexing his neck and upper back. If the pain does not appear to be in the muscle, it should not be treated with massage and the patient should see their doctor if the symptoms persist (see Chapter 12).

Friction can be applied gently along the colon using the knuckles. Rotational movements are made by the wrist as the technique travels in a clockwise direction.

8 Sports Massage

Massage has developed in many directions and we now see several specialized forms of it within a whole spectrum. Sports massage is one specialization that holds a unique position as it has a fundamentally different approach from all other forms of therapy, both orthodox and complementary.

The usual experience in conventional treatment is to aim to restore normal function when someone is injured. But in sport there is no acceptance of 'normal' function in terms of strength, speed or movement. Most athletes hope to reach a level of performance slightly beyond that which they will ever actually achieve. They want to be 'better', not 'normal', and the therapist must also accept this concept. The overall aim of treatment must therefore always be to *enhance performance* at whatever level the sportsman has reached. The most major risk in the quest for enhanced performance is of course injury, so the primary treatment concern is to *prevent injury*.

Sports massage has great potential in this area and this is why many top competitors use it as an integral part of their training regime. With regular treatment they are more able to sustain high levels of performance without getting injured. And the therapist can measure success, not by how well he treats an injury, but by how few actual injuries he has to treat. The great preventative benefits of massage are not yet widely exploited by the recreational sportsman and this is something that needs to be developed through education and greater exposure.

The quality and quantity of training

After a period of hard training or performance there will be an accumulation of waste material and possibly some micro-trauma with slight swelling in the muscles. The tissues will also be nutritionally depleted and some may be in need of repair. By stimulating the blood circulation through the area with massage, all these situations can be helped. The waste is removed more quickly and completely, and more fresh blood from the arteries arrives to supply the repair and nutritional needs.

There should always be a period of rest after hard exercise to allow this recovery process to take place, and massage greatly improves the quality and effectiveness of such rest. It is the quality of rest that is the key to effective training, and regular treatment enables more training at a higher level and with greater safety.

Some athletes may be tempted to take steroids because it is expected to enable them to increase the quality and quantity of their training. Massage could help achieve this safely and legally.

Potential over-use injuries

The most common of all sports injuries is the over-use injury. It can develop slowly over a period of time – days, weeks, months or even years – and the sportsman may not be aware of the problem until it reaches a critical level. As the therapist softens the tissues, these problem areas become apparent as they remain hard and tense compared to the surrounding tissues. Early treatment can prevent this becoming an injury (see Chapter 9).

Training advice

As well as dealing directly with the potential problem, massage also identifies the possibility of a fault in training, which could be causing over-use. It is necessary to compare the condition of the tissues with the individual's training schedule and with any other factors, such as occupation and posture, that could also be relevant. In this way it may be possible to identify very specific components within a training programme that need to be changed or improved. It is common to find a particular muscle that is tight because it is not being effectively stretched, and a correct method can be demonstrated by the therapist to improve this. Other muscles may contain areas of micro-trauma due perhaps to too much strength training. Although these may not be considered an injury at this stage, advice to reduce strength-work for a period or to increase stretching (and massage) can stop it ever becoming one.

Today many people are involved in sport at a competitive level, even though it may be just a recreational activity for them. In many cases they may be performing at a level that 30 years ago would have been considered world-class, or at an age that would then have been unthinkable. They are often doing this without the support and advice of coaches and trainers. Any advice they do get usually comes in the form of tips in magazines and from friends, or through trial and error. The massage therapist may be the only authority on sport and exercise with whom they come into contact, so it is important to give sound advice on any potential problems that may be found.

Self-awareness

Not only will the therapist feel these problems, but so too will the sportsman. Although not previously aware of any problem, he may feel pain in a specific area as deep pressure is applied. When this is done to the same area on the other side of the body, it will probably feel different, and this will make him clearly aware that there is a situation that needs attention.

With improved self-awareness, the sportsman is much more likely to follow the therapist's advice, because it will make real sense. Poor stretching is a common fault, but advice alone is not always enough, because the quality of a stretch is in the 'feel' rather than the position itself. Having felt some pain in the specific area during treatment, the sportsman is acutely aware of where he should feel the stretch and can therefore relax and adjust his position to achieve this.

Fine-tuning

The overall benefit of the advice and self-awareness achieved through sports massage enables the *fine-tuning* of a training programme that is quite unique. However well a programme is devised, it cannot take into account the infinite number of variables that can affect an athlete's life and will influence his susceptibility to injury. Regular sports massage is perhaps the only way to monitor the effects of training on the condition of the tissues. When the athlete, coach and massage therapist work together, regular adjustments can be made to training, which can have a highly positive effect on preventing injury and enhancing performance.

Flexibility

Most sports and all dance activities require good flexibility. Functional stretching exercises should always be performed, not only to promote mobility but also to release excessive tension, fibrosis or scarring in the muscle. But even when done well, exercises may not be fully effective due to restriction in joint range. The elbow joint, for example, cannot extend beyond about 180 degrees, which is not enough to stretch fully all the fibres of the large biceps muscle. Where a problem affects only a small part of a large muscle, the majority of fibres that remain healthy can stretch sufficiently to accommodate the full range without having any effect on the damaged area.

Massage techniques can stretch specific areas of tissue, irrespective of range of movement. Friction and deep stroking techniques can be applied directly to break down scar tissue and adhesions, and can re-align and stretch out very specific areas of damaged or tangled fibres.

Sports injuries

Because most sportsmen continually try to push themselves to new limits, however carefully they train they will inevitably get an injury from time to time. The actual treatment of injury is covered at length throughout this book, but with sport there is a unique difference. The actual treatment of an injury may be the same (regardless of the cause) if the pathology is the same, but the thinking behind the treatment of a sports injury is very different. If someone injuries himself falling off a ladder, it is fair to assume that this will probably be a once-in-a-lifetime experience, which will not happen again. So when it has been success-fully treated it can be forgotten about. But if there is an over-use injury caused by some component in a sports activity, effective treatment alone will not necessarily prevent it recurring. It is vital that any com-ponent in training that may be causing the over-use is identified and changed, to prevent a recurrence of the injury.

In many ways this is the most challenging part of the therapist's work as it requires very careful questioning and a detailed understand-ing of the training methods used.

Common causes of sports injuries

General over-training Doing too much of a particular exercise fatigues the tissues and can cause damage. This should never occur in training, though it often does. But it can easily happen in competition, when the athlete pushes himself to the limit and therefore runs a very real risk of over-exerting. Similarly, problems can arise if training sessions are too frequent, with insufficient time for the tissues to recover fully in between.

Specific over-training This occurs when a particular aspect of training leads to over-use. This can sometimes be the hardest cause to identify as there can be so many possibilities. It could, for example, be just one particular exercise in the gym that is being done incorrectly or that may not be right for that indi-vidual or his sport.

To avoid general over-training, sportsmen often supplement their main activity with other exercise (often called 'cross-training'), which can cause problems if in some small way it conflicts with the demands of the main sport.

A good example of this would be weight training. The best training for a particular sport is actually to do that sport, because the mus-culoskeletal system develops in a balanced way in relation to the demands. But if practised too much, this could lead to general over-use, so the sport is often supplemented with weight training or other gym work that also adds to the particular strengths and skills needed in that sport. However, it is difficult to do this and maintain exactly the right balance of strength and agility. If the main power muscles have been strengthened, it may be possible to perform at a higher level. But if the smaller muscles, which have a secondary or controlling function in the activity, have not also been strengthened, they can become injured because of the increased demands with which they have not been trained to cope. If not directly injured themselves, as they fatigue more quickly their natural movement patterns may become affected and this could lead to other problems.

Specific over-use can also develop when athletes mix the training within their own sport. Endurance athletes, for example, often do some anaerobic training to improve their speed; or sprint athletes do some endurance training to improve their stamina. Using different energy systems, and working the muscles in a way that might not be best suited to them, can cause damage.

Alternative exercise is certainly not a bad thing and is a vital part of many athletes' training schedules, with great possible benefits. But it is important for the therapist to understand that there are potential dangers, which could lead to injury and must be identified in that event so that the right advice can be given.

Warm-up and warm-down This is another area that is commonly neglected, which can result in injury. The particular tissues involved in the activity, as well as the general systems of the body, must be prepared for the stresses they are about to undergo. How this is done is, of course, dependent on the sport in question as well as other factors, such as environment (temperature, weather, etc.). If cold and tight muscles are suddenly expected to expend hard effort they are vulnerable to damage.

A proper warm-down, which again is sport-specific, is also important, as it helps the recovery process to begin properly following hard exercise. After anaerobic activities, for example, maintaining activity at about 50 per cent intensity for a short period is believed to be the best way of facilitating the breakdown of accumulated lactic acid. Stretching is also an important part of a warm-down, as it helps re-align muscle fibres and prevent the natural tightness and stiffness that often follow hard exercise.

Age This may be a relevant factor in relation to the points already mentioned. The ageing process does unfortunately mean that metabolic processes involved in recovery do slow down. And tendons become less well lubricated and so are more prone to damage. There may also be an accumulation of stress on specific structures over many years of repetitive training, leading to wear and tear. The older athlete basically needs to put more effort into helping the natural recovery processes work better. This usually means longer recovery periods (and massage) between training sessions, more stretching and proper warming-up and -down. For athletes who have been in the sport for many years it is often hard to accept these changes and it may be necessary for the therapist to explain the need.

Is it a sports injury? It is easy to assume that if a sportsman has an injury, then it must be a sports injury, but of course this need not be the case. If, for example, a tennis player is complaining of a hip problem, it is better to think first of the whole person, who has a life, family and job, who happens to play tennis and just happens to have a hip problem (see Chapter 10).

Pre- and post-event

Helping an athlete prepare for, and recover from, a competitive event is an important part of sports massage and one that requires a fairly open-minded approach. All athletes have their own unique way of coping, both physically and mentally, with competitive situations, and if this has worked well for them in the past, the therapist should not try to change it with his own ideas.

Pre-event It is important to realize that no two sportsmen respond to massage in quite the same way, and this can present problems if asked to treat an athlete for the first time in a pre-event situation. Ideally, an athlete should see how he responds to pre-event treatment at a competition that is not of major importance to him. This gives both the therapist and the athlete a chance to develop the most suitable procedure.

Pre-event massage can be considered as anything from two days to two minutes before the event, and the treatment approach will differ greatly according to the time-scale. Two days before the event a massage can be deep, thorough and relaxing so that the athlete gets the maximum recuperative benefit from the tapering-down process that should precede an event. Deep treatment, especially if there are specific problem areas to be attended to, may itself take a day or two to recover from and should therefore not be given too close to the event. And deep massage can relax the muscles so much that some athletes find that for a time they lose some of the explosive power they may need.

As the competition gets closer, massage treatment needs to become more specific to the demands of the sport and the wishes of the athlete. The main muscles used in the event are of course the principal ones to treat, and a useful way to find out which these are is to ask the athlete which areas usually tend to hurt most after the event.

It is often assumed that the treatment needs to be stimulating, especially in a sport that requires great speed, strength or explosive power. But pre-competition nervousness and excitement may achieve this anyway and it is sometimes necessary to relax and calm the athlete down a little. This can be done with gentle body rocking and shaking movements rather than by working deeply into the tissues, as the muscles themselves should not be relaxed too much. It is also useful to ask the athlete how he likes to feel generally when he goes into the event. Normally he will want to feel excited and 'fired up', but occasionally you come across an athlete who says he likes to feel more relaxed and 'laid back'. Indeed, there are sports, such as shooting or bowls, where being calm and relaxed is vital for a good performance.

In the last hour or so before an event, massage is not a substitute for a proper warm-up, but should be seen as just one part of the warm-up. For an athlete who is well trained and properly prepared for his event, the effect of the massage at this time should be more psychological than physical and should give an extra boost to his confidence. At this point it may be impractical to use oil, so treatment is usually given through clothing, using shaking, squeezing and pressure techniques.

Working slowly with the techniques will have a relaxing and calming effect, whereas working vigorously will be stimulating. With a sprinter, for example, relaxing the back, neck and shoulders can help prevent these areas from tensing up during the event, or help him stay calm at the start and not jump the gun. At the same time, the legs and lower back can be stimulated as much as possible to help with the explosive power needed to sprint.

Post-event Although most athletes do carry out a warming-down routine after training sessions, they often fail to do so after competition because of sheer exhaustion, elation or perhaps disappointment. Massage can be an adequate substitute for a warm-down as it can achieve much the same effect by removing muscle waste and stretching the tissues.

The method of treatment is the same as with any general sports massage and should be slow and thorough. Care must be taken as there could be some acute problems, so plenty of superficial stroking should be used first to help identify such areas, although the athlete will probably point them out anyway. The treatment of acute inflammation is covered in Chapter 11, but there is a slightly different approach in post-event situations. Ice can be placed on the affected area while massage techniques are applied around and away from it. After a few minutes the ice can be removed and light massage applied over the injured area itself, to dissipate excessive swelling, and then ice can be re-applied. Although any massage is believed to be contraindicated in the acute stage, this method of ice/massage/ice so soon (minutes) after the injury has occurred has been shown to be remarkably effective.

Gentle passive stretching of all the main muscles, or those that feel particularly sore, should be carried out at the end of the massage treatment. This will make up for what the athlete neglects to do, or will add to whatever stretching he has done.

Breaking the rules

On rare occasions a top athlete may sustain a small acute injury immediately before a major event that could be vital to his career, such as an Olympic final. Although, according to the medical 'rule' book, the injury should have a few days' rest and massage is contraindicated, if the *athlete* (not the trainer or anyone else) insists on attempting to compete, then the therapist should do what he can to help.

The therapist can apply a piece of ice on the injury itself, while working with friction and stroking techniques closely around it. The ice can be removed after a few minutes and some light stroking performed over the whole area to improve the lymphatic flow. Ice should be applied again immediately afterwards. Soft Tissue Release (STR, see Chapter 14) is also a very effective technique in this situation. The aim of treatment is to get the best possible function out of the undamaged fibres while speeding up recovery of the damaged ones. There is the obvious risk that working so closely to the injury may increase the damage, but with skill it can produce successful results.

Tapping and strapping will probably be necessary as well, and this should be done by a therapist specifically trained in the method.

9 The Over-Use Syndrome

We use the voluntary muscles of the body to create the movements necessary to conduct our lives, and we should first consider how and why this happens. When we look at a chart of the muscular system for the first time, it is easy to be intimidated by its complexity. There are about 600 skeletal muscles playing their own individual part in moving the body. They are all there for a reason, and if we did not use or need them, then evolution would (or should) over time have caused them to waste away and disappear.

Although the muscular system looks highly complicated, it is important to realize that the actual mechanics involved are very simple. A muscle can do only two things; it can contract (shorten) and relax (lengthen). (It does *not* stretch; it can *be* stretched by the contracting force of opposing muscles or by outside forces such as gravity.) Movement is created by a muscle shortening and so pulling bones together, usually across an articulating joint. So the system is nothing more than a complex pattern made up of many simple levers and pulleys.

The reason for so many muscles is to enable the widest variety of movements and to be able to do them with stability, control and efficiency. If one considers the knee and quadriceps muscles, for example: this is basically a hinge joint capable of moving on only one plane, and so theoretically it should need only *one* pulley to flex it and *one* to extend it. But for extension we have *four* quadriceps muscles, each of which pulls across the joint in a slightly different direction. This stabilizes the joint (along with other structures) and enables it to adapt to variations in movement and to the random direction of forces from the outside environment.

The whole of the muscular system works in unison to enable the body to cope with the stresses caused by gravity (weight) when movement takes place. The running action, for instance, does not just involve the leg muscles. Hundreds of other muscles also work to create a complicated pattern of rotation and spiral movements throughout the entire body. If this did not happen, and movement was confined just to the legs, then all the stress of impact and push-off would be absorbed by the ankle, knee and hip joints, one at a time. The forces would be far too great on these joints individually and they would soon become seriously damaged. The spiralling movement up the body absorbs the stress and distributes the impact through many joints. So no individual structure should absorb too much stress and the human body is therefore able to survive (in gravity) for many years.

It is important to see movement in terms of patterns of activity taking place within a system, rather than as the action of individual muscles. Over-use problems develop in parts of a system that are put under greater stress, or repetitive use, compared to the rest of the system.

The over-use syndrome is most clearly seen in sport, which will be used for the examples here, but many occupational, postural or emotional situations can also have the same effect. All sporting activities have a high repetitive element: cycling is perhaps one of the most extreme examples, where thousands of virtually identical pedal strokes are made. At the other end of the scale something like dance, which entails a wide variety of movements, still involves considerable repetition within a performance as well as in rehearsal.

These repeated movements involve many muscles working together in a pattern to create the power and control needed. As each muscle has a unique function within the system, a particular movement will involve greater effort from certain individual muscles within the pattern. For example, kicking a football involves strong effort from the quadriceps muscles (to extend the knee). Each of the four muscles within the group acts on the joint from a different angle, so depending on the degree of rotation in the lower leg and the angle of the force, one muscle may have to keep working slightly more (or harder) than the rest. A mid-field player who often has to pass the ball with the inside of the foot will tend to use the vastas medialis more. This muscle is made up of numerous bundles of fibres, each of which has its own minutely different action on the muscle as a whole, and so too on the joint. So very small specific areas within a muscle can be put under slightly greater stress than the surrounding tissues. It is here that the over-use syndrome can begin.

Muscle balance or imbalance?

In the above example we would expect the footballer to naturally develop more strength in the vastas medialis as he develops his ability. Although this may appear to create an imbalance with the other quadriceps, it could be natural to the individual and his sport and therefore may not be a situation requiring remedial treatment. If, however, we see the same imbalance in a distance runner who is complaining of knee problems, this could be the key to the problem and would be a treatment priority.

The muscular system develops according to the way we use, over-use or abuse our bodies. Although there are general norms, these are extremely wide and everyone is different. Each individual has his own

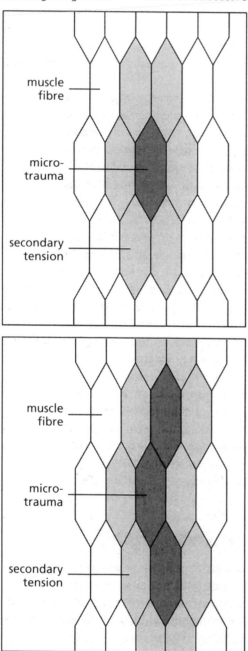

Fig. 1: Micro-trauma affecting a single fibre

Fig. 2: Micro-trauma spreading to adjacent fibres

unique pattern of imbalances, many of which are beneficial and in harmony with his activities and the lifestyle he lives. But some will be negative or excessive. With experience, skill and a degree of intuition, the therapist can work with this in mind and not only treat and prevent minor injury, but also achieve significant postural and functional improvements.

Micro-trauma

We know that a muscle can suffer acute strain, with its fibres being torn, if over-used or overloaded. The same can also occur on a microscopic level if one particular compartment, or in fact just a few fibres within it, are over-used. Although this breakdown occurs on a microscopic level, the pathological changes that take place are just the same as with any soft tissue tear – that is, bleeding and swelling, the onset of secondary muscle tension in the surrounding tissues and the formation of scar tissue (Fig.1). This is what accounts for the general soreness often experienced in muscles after hard exercise: it is due to the high level of micro-trauma and not necessarily to an actual strain (nor the common misconception that it is due to lactic acid).

With any soft tissue strain, rest is vital in the early stages of recovery, but the inflammation caused by micro-trauma may be too small to cause any noticeable pain, so activity may continue with the individual unaware of the problem. A moderate level of exercise is acceptable and may even be quite helpful, as it need only involve the healthy fibres and will promote circulation and prevent adhesions forming in the damaged area. But any greater effort will place a demand on the damaged fibres, which can prevent proper recovery. The scar tissue and tension in and around the micro-trauma prevent any function (contraction or stretching) and so the adjacent fibres have to work harder to make up for this deficiency. These fibres can then become over-used and may also suffer trauma (Fig. 2).

Micro-trauma and scar tissue can then continue to build up gradually, adhesions can form and affect the elasticity within that particular area of the muscle. This in turn makes more of the muscle vulnerable to further micro-trauma, and so the over-use syndrome can develop (Fig. 3).

As function deteriorates in a small part of the muscle, it can create imbalance within the muscle or muscle group, and eventually this can affect the muscular system as a whole. As the condition builds up gradually, in the early stages it may develop unnoticed, and apparently normal activity may continue. The increased tension can then put excessive stress on adjoining structures such as tendons, which can become more vulnerable to acute trauma. Biomechanical faults may develop as natural movement patterns slowly alter, and in the long run the over-use syndrome can lead to many problems, both locally as well as in other parts of the body.

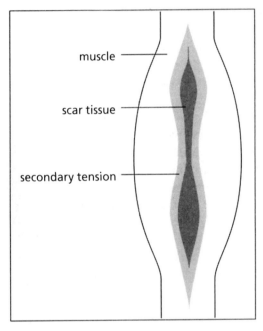

Fig. 3: The over-use syndrome

Massage treatment is possibly the most effective way of identifying this type of problem. It can normally be felt as hardness in a muscle, which usually runs in the same direction as the muscle fibres. Deep transverse stroking is one of the best techniques to use in locating it. The therapist can often feel it long before it actually becomes a painful condition, and so it is probably the most important benefit in general preventative massage. When deep treatment is applied, it will evoke pain, which will make the individual aware of the potential injury problem. In the case of the athlete, this can be a strong inducement to make changes to his training in order to deal with it.

Such areas should be treated in much the same way as any chronic muscle injury, which is just what it is. Friction to break down the scar tissue and stretching to improve flexibility and to re-align tangled fibres are vital for effective treatment. Therapists should look out for signs of micro-trauma and the over-use syndrome during massage as all over-use injuries should be preventable, given the correct early treatment.

Any over-use injury that has occurred once will probably recur if the same activity, or level of activity, is repeated. It is therefore important always to try and find the specific aspect of activity, or component in sport, that may be causing the over-use. To do this successfully requires experience more than anything else. It is necessary to compare the conditions you find in the tissues with what you know of how the individual uses his body. Sports activity or occupation alone may not provide all the answers, as postural or environmental factors may also be involved.

Although we usually associate over-use in terms of active movement, inactivity can sometimes lead to similar problems. Computer keyboard operators, for example, commonly suffer occupational stress problems due to a fixed posture and lack of movement. The body is capable of a huge variety of movements and activities, but does not cope well with staying in an almost fixed position for long periods of time. The common position often adopted when working at a keyboard involves a continual shortening of the upper trapezius and posterior neck muscle, to raise the shoulders and hold the head up from a forward leaning position. This puts stress on specific tissues, causing micro-trauma in a similar way to the active type of over-use. Lack of movement in the muscles also slows the blood-flow through the area, which can increase congestion and add to the problem.

Another factor concerning the over-use syndrome in occupational/postural situations is that stretching a tight muscle causes mild discomfort. The body instinctively avoids this uncomfortable sensation by involuntarily raising the shoulders even higher, which in turn increases tension in the long run. This process happens on a level that we are not consciously aware of. Often no discomfort at all is felt until it reaches a critical level of tension and function becomes noticeably affected, or perhaps a sudden movement or bad sleeping position causes spasm or strain.

A common example is the patient who appears to have done nothing out of the ordinary but wakes up one morning with a stiff neck. The normal, healthy body will not suddenly go wrong for no reason – there has to be an over-use factor involved.

10 Other Stress Factors

All injuries must have a cause. Sometimes this is obvious, as in the case of accidental injuries, where external forces can easily be identified. Other injuries, however, may *appear* to have an obvious cause, especially in sport, where a particular activity brings on painful symptoms. But if it was purely due to the activity, then everyone who did that activity could expect to get the same injury. If ten athletes complete an event at the same level, why does only one suffer from the injury? Why do all computer keyboard operators not suffer the same neck and shoulder problems? There must be other precipitating factors involved, which add to the patient's susceptibility to injury, in addition to the activity itself. There are also some injuries that seem, to the patient, to occur without any identifiable cause at all. But a healthy body does not suddenly self-distruct without a reason. Again, there must be some contributory factor involved.

Although this chapter deals with different stress factors, these are not mutually exclusive. They all interrelate with each other and, to a greater or lesser degree, could all be involved in every injury situation.

Posture

A particular action may result in injury to one person rather than another due to postural factors. Restriction or dysfunction in one area may cause specific tissues elsewhere to be overloaded and injured, as they have to work harder to compensate. For example, a restriction in the lower back can cause over-use in the upper back. Or a misalignment of the shoulder can lead to over-use in a specific muscle involved in its action.

Rarely will a patient have a perfectly balanced posture, and even if this is not contributing to an injury, it can still have a negative effect on general health and well-being. So even in a general massage situation, where a specific injury is not involved, there will always be some degree of imbalance that can be worked upon and improved.

Posture is primarily determined by hereditary factors, such as bone structure, muscle type and even by habitual movement patterns. These can create natural imbalances, but these alone do not normally lead to painful conditions until later life. They can, however, combine with other stresses and together can lead to injury. Little can be done actually to change these hereditary factors, and regular exercise and treatment are often the only way of avoiding such symptoms.

Much of our posture is acquired through the way we use our body and develop the muscles. As such, it is always changing and adapting. At the end of a day posture may deteriorate and become more slumped, as the muscles fatigue through work and effort. In the long term,

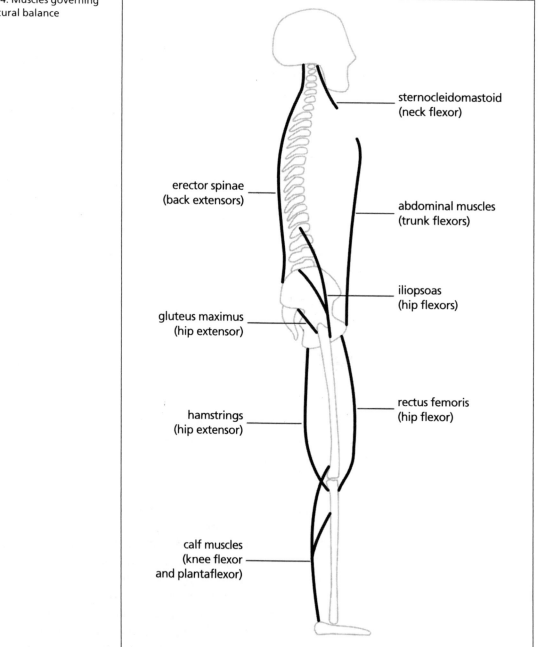

Fig. 4: Muscles governing postural balance

sternocleidomastoid
(neck flexor)

erector spinae
(back extensors)

abdominal muscles
(trunk flexors)

iliopsoas
(hip flexors)

gluteus maximus
(hip extensor)

rectus femoris
(hip flexor)

hamstrings
(hip extensor)

calf muscles
(knee flexor
and plantaflexor)

general trends in the daily fatigue patterns can have a cumulative effect, which gradually changes posture more permanently.

Occasional injury situations can cause short-term postural changes, due to local areas of pain and dysfunction, as well as through compensation. Although this should return to normal after the injury has recovered, postural imbalances often remain and these can add to the other permanent changes taking place.

Upright posture is maintained by a series of muscles running down the front and back of the body (Fig. 4). These need to balance each other, in terms of strength and tension, and together resist the forces of gravity. Any postural change will nearly always be in a downward direction, as fatigue or injury reduces the ability of the postural muscles to combat gravity. This creates increased curvature in particular sections of the spine, which can be seen by the therapist when observing the patient's standing posture.

Common postural imbalances

Cervical lordosis
- Tight or strong upper erector spinae. This is usually a postural compensation for a thoracic curvature and the sternocleidomastoid muscles may not be weak, although they may shorten and become tense.

Thoracic kyphosis
- Weak erector spinae
- Tight abdominals and sternocleidomastoid

Lumbar lordosis
- Tight lower erector spinae
- Weak abdominals

Forward-tilting pelvis (almost always associated with a lumbar lordosis)
- Tight gluteus maximus and rectus femoris
- Weak abdominals and iliopsoas

Backward-tilting pelvis
- Tight hip extensors, abdominals, iliopsoas and hamstrings
- Weak rectus femoris

Sway-back knees
- Tight calf muscles and rectus femoris
- Weak hamstrings

None of these will occur in isolation as an imbalance in one area will generally lead to imbalances developing in adjacent areas as they compensate.

Only the posterior/anterior posture is considered here, but distortions can occur in lateral and rotational directions, too. These will involve imbalance between the postural muscles on either side of the body, and also reciprocal imbalances in some of the voluntary muscles of the torso.

Muscle imbalance leads to problems in the bone structure, and structural bone problems will lead to muscle imbalance. Both need to be attended to, and although the massage therapist cannot directly treat the bone structures, working with the muscles alone can have a great effect.

There is no single answer to these postural problems. Significant improvements usually require a variety of specialized skills to rectify muscle balance, structural alignment and freedom and, most importantly, function. Without improving function the patient will not fully utilize the structural freedom created by massage or other therapies, and so the imbalances may return.

Environment

The general environment within which we live and work can involve unduly high levels of stress and these can have a direct effect on the structure of the body and can contribute to injury. Great mental demand and worry can all drain energy and lead to muscular fatigue and tension. Even a poor environment, such as cold, damp, noise or disturbed sleep, can add to the physical stress of daily life.

Any aspects of a patient's life may play a part in contributing to an injury situation. Although it is not the role of the massage therapist to deal with these matters, it is important to accept that they exist. Sometimes during general conversation between patient and therapist a stress factor of this nature may emerge. The therapist can advise the patient that this may be contributing to his injury, and the patient can then take action himself to deal with it.

Psycho/emotional factors

Psychology and emotion play a part in all aspects of life and injury is no exception. In some clinical situations, despite good and apparently effective treatment, the patient continues to suffer painful symptoms. And some patients seem to suffer continually from one injury or another. Although there may be physical or medical reasons for this, underlying psychological factors may also be influencing the situation. Although this is not an area in which the massage therapist should attempt to work, it is important to be aware of the possibility of these factors.

Holding on to injury A patient will sometimes hold on to an injury because it satisfies other needs. He will usually have had the problem for a long time and will have been to other therapists before. Although treatment may not identify any significant tissue damage, the patient will still experience pain. He may be holding on to the injury because:

- If he feels socially or emotionally insecure, the injury gives him support and sympathy from the people around him.
- It gives him the excuse to avoid activities in which he has a fear of failure, or situations where he feels he has poor social skills.
- It makes a good excuse for poor performance.
- Continuing in his sport or activity, despite his pain, makes him appear to be a martyr.

It is important to accept that the pain the patient feels is usually quite real, and to say that there is not a problem would be quite wrong. Although the massage therapist should not attempt to deal with the psychological aspect of the injury without proper training, by being a sympathetic listener he can sometimes help the patient see the problem for himself.

Massage treatment alone may give slight improvement in the symptoms for a few treatments, but then the patient usually moves on to another therapist and starts again.

Emotional factors   Painful injury is sometimes the physical symptom of an underlying emotional problem. This will tend to concern a very major issue in life, which the patient is unwilling, or unable, to confront.

Some true cases:

- A patient had been off work for six months due to a chronic lower back injury. He had extensive treatment, including surgery, and was considered to have recovered fully. The painful symptoms in his back began to return by lunchtime on his first day back at the office. Surprisingly though, he enjoyed his job. It was living in London that he hated and he wanted to return to his home territory. The job was tying him to London and perhaps he was trying to force himself through the injury to give it up.

- A sportsman with a minor calf injury that had troubled him for two years found that it miraculously went away, never to return, the day after he and his wife agreed to a divorce!

- After suffering from minor lower backache for four years, a patient received deep massage treatment for the first time. Over the next few days he felt very emotional and kept thinking about his dead father. His back problem recovered very quickly and never returned. He had not experienced much grief when his father died four years before, and his back problem had begun about three months later.

Psychology of injury in sport

Pre-competition   Some sportsmen tend to suffer injuries just before major competition. Sometimes the injury itself may be quite minor, but the patient's perception of the pain and discomfort can be very great. It is possible that this is due to fear of the public assessment of his performance and a potential failure to do well.

Over-training Some sportsmen regularly suffer injuries due to continual over-training. Even though logically they know it makes sense, they will be reluctant to cut down and will ignore advice to do so. The injuries are perhaps just a symptom of their desire to achieve too much in their sport. Or they may be putting all their effort and attention into their sport to avoid having to confront a more serious personal issue in their life.

11 Acute and Post-Acute Injuries

Acute treatment

A *strain* to a muscle or tendon is probably the most common type of acute injury. This occurs when the tissue fibres become torn or damaged and causes bleeding and swelling, due to overloading or stretching. As well as pain and dysfunction, heat and redness may be noticed with injuries that occur near the surface.

The other common injury is the joint *sprain,* where a ligament that supports the joint is torn. This occurs if a joint is forced beyond its normal range, especially when load-bearing. The symptoms here are usually much more noticeable than with a strain as there is considerable swelling and bruising, and much pain and dysfunction with any attempt to put movement or pressure through the joint.

Ideally, these injuries should be attended to immediately by a qualified therapist, but this is hardly ever the case because of the location at the time. This should not be a problem as everything that needs to be done can easily be self-administered. Many books explain how to treat acute injuries, but the general public never seems to read them until it is too late. All too often people try to do what they think is best, based on their general knowledge. And with the best intentions they usually get it about half right and three-quarters wrong, because they do the right things the wrong way.

As well as being vital that the therapist knows how to treat acute conditions, it is also his duty to educate the patient. Acute injuries rarely happen when a therapist is present, so he must know how to act correctly himself or be able to help an injured colleague. (Print a leaflet and give it to all your patients.)

Follow the RICE (Rest, Ice, Compression, Elevation) procedure for the first 24–48 hours (depending on the severity) after the injury.

Rest Rest for the injured area is absolutely vital in this early stage. If fibres have been torn apart, any movement will continue to open and aggravate the tear and cause much more bleeding. Immediate rest from any movement or load-bearing enables the fibres to begin to knit together quickly before any more damage is done. It is far better to over-react with too much rest in the early stage than to try and ignore the symptoms. The temptation to try and use the injured part, to see if it still hurts, *must* be avoided during this initial period. No real fitness will be lost in just two days, but if the trauma is aggravated it could take much longer in the end to get back to normal activity.

Ice   Ice should be applied as soon as possible, as this slows down blood circulation and so reduces the amount of bleeding and swelling in the tissues. If ice is not available, anything cold will do, although 'cold sprays' are often only effective on superficial injuries and so are not really much use with most large traumas. For the spray to cool the deeper tissues it would have to be applied for so long that the skin would be damaged (frozen). The method of spraying for intermittent periods may prevent this but it is labour-intensive. Cold packs are the easy, cheap and effective option. Ice should not be placed directly on the skin as this can cause it to burn. The ice should be wrapped in a wet cloth, which prevents this and also acts as a good heat conductor. Ice can, however, be applied directly to the skin if it is kept moving slowly and smoothly over the general area as it melts. Using a balm or anti-inflammatory ointment on the skin helps the ice glide along and seems to create an even better effect.

Ice should only be applied locally to the injury site and, if dealing with a limb injury, it should not go all the way round it as this will restrict blood-flow to the more distal parts. One error often made is in the timing of this treatment, because if ice is applied for too long it can make the problem worse. Instead of slowing the circulation, the defence mechanism of the body reverses this and begins to send more blood to the area to prevent the skin from freezing. This can increase the bleeding and swelling. How long ice is applied for depends mainly on the area involved – a small area like the wrist will chill much more quickly (about 5 minutes) than a large area like the thigh (up to 20 minutes). To help judge the right amount of time, observe the colour of the skin: if it looks red when the ice is removed, it means it was too long; ideally the skin should look pale. Ice treatment (cryotherapy) can be repeated often, providing enough time is given to allow the skin temperature to return to normal before repeating it. It is particularly important to try to re-ice the area if it is aggravated by any accidental (or otherwise) activity using that part of the body.

Reducing circulation is the common reason given for icing an acute injury, but this may not be the only advantage. If the area is properly rested, the fibres will close very quickly and bleeding will stop naturally anyway. The ice, however, does have an analgesic effect, by chilling and numbing the pain receptors and inhibiting sensory nerve conductivity. By reducing the pain sensation it also reduces the protective spasm around the injury, and the area becomes more relaxed. This allows the swelling to dissipate more quickly and the healing process to begin.

Compression   Compression should be applied to the area as immediately as possible to restrict bleeding at the injury site. The pressure compresses the blood vessels, so preventing blood from escaping through the open ends of the torn fibres. Compression should be applied by using a firm pad over the injury site, with a strapping around it to hold it in place. Do not apply compression around a whole limb, as this will starve other areas of blood.

Elevation Elevation of the injured area should be practised as much as possible. A leg or arm should be comfortably supported so that it is raised higher than the torso. This allows gravity to assist the removal of swelling from the area and so aids recovery.

Correct and immediate acute treatment as described here can achieve fantastic results and, if carried out immediately, can remove the symptoms of the injury almost completely. Although pain may be much reduced, damaged fibres are still in the very early stage of repair and can easily be re-damaged. It is important to emphasize the continued need to rest the area, even though pain may be minimal, and the temptation to test it to see if it still hurts must be resisted.

All acute injuries should (ideally) be seen by a medical practitioner as soon as possible. But as the majority of strains and sprains are quite minor, the inflammation soon stops and the patient may choose not to seek other medical help. However, if the area remains inflamed after 48 hours, despite good RICE procedure, this suggests that it could be more than a minor soft tissue injury and must be medically assessed.

Massage Massage should not be applied directly to an acute injury because the movement that it will create within the tissues can re-open the tears in the fibres. And, by increasing the circulation, it will also encourage more bleeding. However, general massage techniques away from the injury, to improve lymphatic drainage, are very beneficial and can be given at the same time as the RICE procedure.

Post-acute treatment

Treatment in the post-acute phase of a trauma is harder to explain, because so much depends on the particular nature and location of it. When the signs of inflammation have gone and swelling, heat and redness are much reduced (usually after about 48 hours) the MICE (Mobilization, Ice, Compression, Elevation) procedure should be followed.

Mobilization Mobilization (sometimes called 'active' rest) is the key to a full and speedy recovery. There should be a gradual and progressive introduction of exercise over a period of time.

This can begin with active movements, with the patient taking the injured part through its full pain-free range without any weight or resistance. Not only does this work the muscles and so prevent atrophy, but it also shows the therapist the safe range to work within. After three or four days the patient should be encouraged to try and gently start to actively increase this range, within pain tolerance.

Passive movements can be performed on the patient by the therapist, who can slowly move the part through its pain-free range. It is important to give firm, comfortable support and to get the patient to relax and co-operate in this. Protective muscle contraction often occurs spontaneously to prevent a movement that the body 'thinks' will cause pain. These gentle, passive movements give the body 'reassurance' that more normal movement can be made without danger and the need for this protection. At the limits of the pain-free range, passive stretches can be applied very gently to prevent (or release) fibrous adhesions and to increase the functional range.

As the injury recovers, exercises with resistance can be introduced. Isometric exercises are good in the early stages, particularly with joint injuries. The therapist fixes the area in a comfortable position and the patient attempts to move it in all directions against the fixed resistance. This can also be done the other way round, with the patient keeping the joint fixed as the therapist tries to move it in all directions. As no movement takes place, the joint will not be put at any risk but the associated muscles will be stimulated by the exercise.

To restore strength, resistance needs to be applied throughout the active range. This can initially be done with the therapist offering minimal resistance and allowing the patient to work through the range of which he is capable. It is important to concentrate on the range and quality of movement first, using light pressure, and to encourage the patient to take it as far as possible. Once good range has been restored, stronger resistance can be used to restore strength.

When basic function has been regained there can be a gradual and controlled return to a normal level of activity. In the case of a runner with a leg injury, for example, he needs to be able to go for a brisk walk first, then try jogging, and only when this can be done without difficulty should he attempt to run.

If pain is experienced at the injury site during exercise, the activity should be stopped. If the pain disappears in 20–30 seconds, then exercise can continue with caution as this may only have been a protective muscle spasm. If the pain persists, then stop and rest for 24 hours, following the RICE procedure, before resuming exercise at an easier level.

Ice Ice treatment should be continued for up to about a week, especially if there is any discomfort following mobilization exercises.

Heat, in the form of infra-red lamps or hot pads, can be used after four to five days, providing inflammation has stopped. Heat helps promote healing by stimulating circulation but should not be applied for more than half an hour at a time, as metabolism suffers if heated for too long.

Contrast baths, or alternating between hot and cold baths for one minute at a time, is another method that can be extremely effective. As well as stimulating the circulation, the contrasting sensory nerve stimulation can be highly relaxing and can release muscle tension.

Compression Compression should be continued for a few days, then gradually reduced to just a support bandage as the condition improves. There are specific taping and strapping techniques that allow activity to resume while offering protection to the damaged tissues.

Elevation Elevation of the injured part should be done as often as possible until all swelling has gone.

Massage Lymphatic drainage techniques (see below) should be used until the swelling has gone down. Gentle, superficial stroking techniques can be applied directly to strains and sprains, usually after about three days. Deeper stroking and light friction can usually be started after about five days. Treatment should not cause too much pain (though some discomfort is inevitable), otherwise it may be causing further damage. The aim of massage is to:

- Reduce swelling
- Stimulate circulation (promote healing)
- Prevent excessive scar tissue forming
- Prevent, or break down, adhesions

Lymphatic drainage massage

The good functioning of the lymphatic system is of paramount importance in acute injury as its main function is to reduce the swelling. The accumulation of fluid and damaged cell particles needs to be removed quickly from the injured area to promote good recovery.

As lymph vessels have little pressure, the flow is affected more by gravity and the primary pumping force comes from muscle activity. With acute injuries there is an increased demand on the system to drain the area, but the muscle activity needed to achieve this is unfortunately reduced because of the pain and dysfunction. All forms of massage will stimulate the flow of lymph as it pumps the circulation towards the heart. But when dealing with a particular area of swelling it is necessary to take a more specific approach.

The injured area should be comfortably supported in a well-elevated position. If the injury is in the distal part of a limb, it is necessary to clear the lymph vessels in the proximal area first. This can be done with basic deep stroking techniques, working towards the lymph nodes in the groin and armpit areas. Pressure should only be applied as the stroke goes away from the injury and there should be nothing more than skin contact as the hand returns to perform the next stroke. Treatment can gradually move towards the injury, using short pumping strokes as well as long strokes. Pressure should be reduced when getting close to the area to avoid disturbing the tissues and causing pain. Return several times to pump the system in the proximal part of the limb to clear the vessels there so that they can cope with the fluid being moved from the injury site.

12 Musculoskeletal Injuries

In the overall treatment of injury, massage does have limitations. It can only be used directly to treat the soft tissues, and only those that can actually be reached by the palpating hand. And where damage is quite major, more advanced forms of treatment than massage may be required to facilitate the initial repair. The therapist should therefore only see himself in an independent role when dealing with minor soft tissue problems. These are the most common of all injuries and often do not get adequately dealt with in a busy modern health service. Despite the limitations of massage, however, there is huge demand for the therapist's skill in treating such minor injuries.

Ideally the decision about the severity of the injury and the best form of treatment to use should be made by a medical practitioner, but this may not always be the case. The massage therapist therefore also needs to be able to assess a situation (but *not* to diagnose the condition) in terms of its soft tissue component. Where the soft tissues appear to be the primary cause of the problem and the damage is relatively minor, although pain and dysfunction may be considerable, the massage therapist can proceed in treating it. Should symptoms fail to improve after two or three sessions, however, underlying factors should be considered and the patient referred to a doctor, physiotherapist or osteopath for their opinion.

Any injury that appears to involve more serious damage to the soft tissues, or where there may be bone or articular damage, must be referred to a more senior practitioner. Massage may still form part of the treatment, as there will always be a soft tissue component to attend to, but it may need to be carried out under medical supervision. Whether the massage therapist is working independently on a minor condition or in association with a more senior practitioner, the basic treatment procedure is the same whatever the type of soft tissue involved.

General procedures with soft tissue inflammation (see also Chapter 3)

The acute stage Massage is locally contraindicated and the therapist should ensure that good acute treatment (RICE) procedures are used. General massage can be applied elsewhere and away from the injury site to reduce swelling and prevent secondary problems developing. By following the correct procedures inflammation should stop within 24–48 hours.

The post-acute stage When there are no longer any signs of inflammation and swelling has reduced, massage of the injury site can begin. It should start with gentle stroking and kneading to stimulate the circulation, reduce swelling and generally mobilize the superficial tissues. Gentle friction can also be applied to prevent scar tissue forming into adhesions with adjacent fibres or structures. Easy mobilization techniques should also be introduced at this stage to help prevent further muscular imbalances developing.

Chronic inflammation Where a low level of inflammation has continued for a considerable time, or a large trauma in the past has not been given good treatment, there may be a considerable build-up of scar tissue with a large area of congested fibrous tissue in and around the injury site. This needs to be treated with much deeper friction in order to break it down, and deep longitudinal strokes will help to re-align the fibres.

During rehabilitation Deep massage can be applied with friction into the damaged area. This will break down excessive scar tissue, continue the benefits of increased circulation and improve tissue mobility. Active and resisted mobilization techniques can be used within reasonable limits of pain (see also Chapter 16).

It is always important to include deep treatment to all the muscles and other soft tissue associated with the injury site. The root cause, or contributing factors, may be found there and/or secondary problems may develop in these tissues.

Bone injuries

Fractures Bones can be fractured as a result of extreme stress, which is usually associated with a fall or impact. People usually know when they have a possible bone fracture and will normally go to a hospital first, but this may not always be the case.

Symptoms
- Pain and tenderness around the injury site caused by movement or weight-bearing
- Swelling and bruising in the injured area due to associated soft tissue damage
- Deformity and abnormal movement in the fractured bone

In certain circumstances these symptoms may not be obvious, such as with fractures in the neck or foot, or where a compression force impacts the fracture, making it remain fairly stable. If the circumstances of the injury suggest the possibility of a fracture, then a referral should always be considered.

Full repair usually takes about six weeks for an upper limb and up to 12 weeks for a lower limb, but sometimes can take much longer, especially in older patients. The soft tissues around the fracture normally get damaged too and the scar tissue that this creates can easily form adhesions because of the immobilization needed during the initial recovery. Deep friction massage is therefore very important to help restore soft tissue function as soon as the bone has repaired sufficiently to take the pressure.

Stress fractures
These usually occur as a result of a repeated load over a long period of time. They are most likely to surface in activities involving repetitive impact on hard surfaces, such as distance running, tennis or ballet. The tibia and fourth and fifth metatarsal bones are those most commonly affected.

The body adapts to training over time, so bones will gradually become thicker and stronger to enable them to cope with a particular stress. A marathon runner with 10 years' experience may be able to maintain a training schedule of over 100 miles/160 km per week, but if someone tried to reach that level in only two years it could result in a stress fracture, because the bones might not yet be strong enough to cope. On a shorter time-scale, whenever there is a rapid increase in training and/or a sudden introduction of a high stress component in training, there is the increased risk of a stress fracture.

Fatigue theory
During repeated, extreme training the muscles pass their peak of endurance and are not fully able to support the structure during impact. The load is therefore transferred into the skeleton rather than being absorbed by the muscles. If this load exceeds the tolerance of the bone, a stress fracture may occur.

Overload theory
Some muscle groups contract in such a way as to cause a bending of the bone. The calf muscles, for example, cause the tibia to bend when they contract. Continual bending over a sustained period can cause a stress fracture.

Symptoms
Stress fractures are difficult to diagnose without advanced imaging equipment, and the physical symptoms can sometimes be vague.

- Symptoms may come on gradually, or suddenly, without any apparent trauma.
- In the early stage symptoms may be felt when exercising but not at rest. Later they become more acute with exercise and ache when at rest.
- Local pain and swelling can usually be felt over the fracture site.

Normally X-rays will only identify stress fractures when they can pick up the formation of scar tissue after about three or four weeks. Modern scanning methods are better, but not as readily available.

One simple, but fairly effective, way to assess the possibility of a stress fracture is to relax the soft tissues by holding the part in a neutral position. Take a firm grip of the two ends of the bone and wiggle it slowly and progressively in different directions. If a localized pain is felt along the shaft of the bone, this is a strong indication of a stress fracture.

Rest is the only way to allow the bone to heal after a stress fracture, although it is claimed that some electrotherapy machines can accelerate the healing process.

Periosteum (periostitis) The periosteum membrane lines the bone and forms the attachment with the tendons. It may become inflamed due to repetitive stress, which tends to occur at the tendon attachment (tenoperiostitis). The problem usually occurs in association with muscle/tendon injuries, making it difficult to identify.

Typically these injuries affect the lower leg and are more likely to occur in people who train on hard surfaces or work with heavy weights. The medial border of the tibia is the most common site of these injuries (so-called 'shin splints') and also around the calcaneum bone, where the Achilles tendon attaches.

The condition can become chronic as it is often difficult for the leg to be given sufficient rest for proper recovery. Scar tissue may build up along the surface of the bone, making it feel ragged and uneven. Although massage to the surrounding area will aid recovery in post-acute conditions, friction should be used cautiously as it may cause more inflammation (ice can be applied after treatment to try and prevent this).

Joint injuries

Dislocation Total dislocations (luxation) most commonly occur to the shoulder, elbow, finger or patella joints. Partial dislocations (subluxation) are more likely at the knee, ankle and acromioclavicular joint. They are caused by the bones of the joint being forced out of their normal location.

The symptoms are usually obvious, with considerable pain, dysfunction and deformity. Relocation of the joint by a medical practitioner should be carried out immediately. The quicker this happens, the shorter the recovery time will be.

All joints are surrounded by a synovial capsule and other soft tissues, which also get damaged when a dislocation occurs. After relocation of the bones, this will need to be attended to with massage techniques, in the usual way.

Ligament injuries

Sprain Ligaments may tear if a joint is forced beyond its normal range, either because of too great a force, or through sudden movement, which is too rapid for the proprioceptive system to respond to. As the ligaments control the range of joint movement, and so protect the bone structures, there is the possibility of bone damage with a major tear, and medical assessment may need to be considered.

Partial or complete tears may occur anywhere along the ligament. Occasionally the ligament may tear at the insertion and break a small piece of bone off with it (avulsion fracture). Even with minor sprains there will be considerable bleeding into the joint, resulting in much swelling and bruising. During the acute phase it is vital that the joint is rested, and fixed so that the damaged ligament is in a slightly shortened position. Without this the tear might be held open and fibrous tissue will form in the gap, resulting in a permanently loose ligament that will not support the joint properly.

Acute sprains often turn into chronic conditions due to a build-up of scar tissue and adhesions, usually because of inadequate treatment in the early stage. This can lead to the ligament becoming thick and inflexible and adhering to other structures. It may become permanently too short or too long, depending on the way it is misused during early repair. With poor recovery, the joint may remain unstable and can easily be re-injured. Along with massage treatment, remedial exercises are very important to help restore good, stable function.

To test for ligament damage, the joint should be passively moved by the therapist. There should be no pain through its inner range, but a fairly sudden onset of pain will be felt as it reaches the end of its free range. If the therapist can feel only a soft resistance at this position, and when a gentle isometric contraction in the opposite direction does not cause an increase in pain, then the ligament is the most likely structure involved.

Inner articular structures

Damage or inflammation of the articular surfaces or inner joint structures can usually be identified by compressing the bones together and/or gliding them across one another. And when passively moving the joint there may be a feeling of a hard resistance, as well as pain, at the end of the free range.

Inflammation or damage to the articular surfaces are dealt with under Arthritis in Chapter 17.

The knee joint has two important cruciate ligaments running through the centre of it (crossing posterior/anterior between the femur and tibia). If damaged, gliding the tibia back and forth across the femur may not always reproduce the painful symptoms but will show more laxity compared with the other knee. It is impossible to reach these structures directly with massage and so other procedures are necessary.

Bursae (bursitis)

Bursae are small fluid-filled sacs that act as cushions, reducing friction and distributing stress. They are usually found around joints and are located between tissues like bone and tendon, tendon and tendon, or tendon and overlying skin.

They can become inflamed if irritated by rubbing or by being compressed against other tissues. Tight tendons can do this as they pull harder across the joint, or the bones may irritate them through repetitive joint movement in an extreme range. Both of these situations become more likely if there is also poor joint alignment. Peripheral joints are more susceptible to damage through impact or external pressure, which can also cause inflammation. ('Housemaid's knee' is inflammation of the infrapatellar bursa, usually caused by kneeling on hard surfaces.)

Pain is usually referred generally into the joint area and it is difficult to distinguish bursitis from other soft tissue injury, especially as they often occur together. In mild conditions, normal massage procedures, along with rest, are usually very effective.

Acquired bursae can form just under the skin in areas that are subject to constant pressure, or where acute impact trauma may have occurred in the past. These may not cause any pain but can be unsightly and, if in close proximity to a joint, may restrict movement. Deep friction is highly effective in breaking them down.

Loose bodies

Small particles of dense material can form within the joint capsule and may float around inside it. They are often made up of pieces of ligament or tendon, which have flaked or broken away from their main structure. If they become lodged between articulating or moving structures, they can cause restriction and become an irritant, which leads to inflammation. Symptoms tend to come and go fairly randomly without any obvious precipitating factors.

Massage treatment will be of variable success with loose bodies. Sometimes it may dislodge the particle and move it somewhere it can do less harm. At other times friction may cause further inflammation by irritating the tissues around it.

Symptomatic joint pain

It is the muscles that make a joint move, and many apparent joint problems are due to dysfunction or imbalance in these muscles. They can cause the joint to function incorrectly and pain may be experienced there and not in the affected muscles. A weak muscle can affect the free movement of the joint and lead to other tissues becoming damaged. A tight muscle can pull more forcefully on its attachment, causing micro-trauma as well as affecting movement.

Dysfunction in a joint will cause problems to develop quite quickly in the associated muscles; and dysfunction in the muscles can eventually cause problems in the joint. The primary and secondary conditions are interlinked and both must be attended to, to achieve good results.

The muscular component of a joint condition can be assessed through active and passive movements. If the muscle is tight, weak or otherwise damaged, the joint pain is more likely to develop gradually as it is passively stretched towards the end of its free range. If it is isometrically contracted in this position, the pain will usually increase. Strong muscle contraction within the free range may also reproduce the painful joint symptoms.

Chronic joint pain

With conditions that have developed over a long period of time, the problem is rarely isolated to just one structure. A small area of damage that restricts joint function will often lead to associated tissues becoming over-used as they try to make up for the deficiency. Eventually many small areas of scar tissue and fibrous adhesions may develop around the joint structures, causing general pain and dysfunction.

The joint must be palpated thoroughly to find and treat all the tissues contributing to the problem. It should be moved into different positions so that the therapist can gain access to as many tissues and surfaces as possible.

Muscle injuries

Strain (also called a tear or rupture) The most common of all injuries is the muscle strain. Muscle movement is the principal factor in all physical activity, especially sport, so it is understandable that muscles get injured so often. Most strains are fairly minor and are often not seen by a medical practitioner. But without good treatment even minor strains may repair poorly and result in permanent scarring and adhesions in the tissues, which will impair function.

Direct trauma (compression rupture) occurs when direct impact causes rupture and bleeding in the muscle, and it is obviously more common in contact sports or accidental injury. Such traumas may occur at a very deep level if fibres become damaged by being compressed against the underlying bone.

Indirect trauma (distraction rupture) can be caused by overload, overstretch or by a shearing force, and is common in activities involving explosive muscle activity. Athletes are more prone to this if they have a poor stretching and warm-up programme, or if the tissues are cold. The rupture occurs when the demand is greater than the strength or elasticity of the muscle, and the fibres become torn as the force exceeds their contractile strength. The symptoms of such strains often come on suddenly with an acute injury, but in minor cases they may not be felt until the next day.

Over-use strain can develop more slowly in activities that have a high repetitive element, with occupation and sport being the usual examples. The symptoms may build up slowly into a chronic condition without there necessarily being an acute stage (see also Chapter 9).

Partial ruptures (first degree) involve up to 5 per cent of the muscle fibres. There is only a minor loss of strength and function, but active or passive movements will cause some pain. *Partial ruptures* (second degree) involve more fibres, and there is pain with any attempt to contract the muscle. *Total ruptures* (third degree) involve a complete tearing of the whole muscle. No functional movement is possible, as there is no longer any connection with the bone. Total ruptures must be seen by a medical practitioner as soon as possible. Immediate surgical repair is sometimes the only way to achieve a good recovery.

Symptoms
- A sharp, stabbing pain may be felt at the time the injury occurs, and afterwards there is pain when the muscle tries to contract. Pain may cause a protective spasm, which further inhibits function. At rest there may be only a little pain caused by the pressure of the swelling.
- With a partial rupture it may be possible to feel a lump in the muscle, where the torn fibres became bunched up as they recoiled from the tear, and a gap may be felt in the adjacent tissues.
- With a total rupture, a large lump will be felt where the whole muscle bunches up.
- Local pain and swelling will occur due to bleeding.
- Bruising may appear after 24 hours but not necessarily directly over the injury site as the blood may track through other tissues before nearing the surface.

When muscle fibres tear, their natural elasticity causes them to recoil, which leaves a space. This fills with blood, which contains all the ingredients necessary for healing. The repair of the injury involves two factors: the formation of new muscle fibres (regeneration) and the simultaneous production of scar tissue. Skeletal muscle has a good regenerating capacity, but the key factor governing recovery is the amount of bleeding that also occurs from the blood vessels that get torn at the same time (haematoma). Under some circumstances, relatively minor strains may result in a greater amount of haematoma due to poor acute treatment, and so may take longer to recover than a more serious strain that is properly dealt with at the time. During exercise there is a considerable re-distribution of blood-flow as the circulation to the working muscles increases. If fibres tear in these muscles during exercise there will be considerably greater haematoma, especially if the activity continues instead of immediately resting the muscle.

Intramuscular haematoma Strains may occur within the muscle sheath (fascia), and the damage and bleeding will be contained within that compartment. If the fascia has not also been torn, the blood is less able to escape from the area and so considerable intramuscular pressure can build up. In the acute stage this is perhaps beneficial, as the pressure compresses blood vessels and so restricts further bleeding to some extent. But it may also impair recovery in the post-acute stage, because a good blood supply is needed for repair. Without proper treatment this type of strain may result in a large build-up of scar tissue, adhesions and fibrosis deep within the muscle. It can also sometimes lead to compartment syndrome due to increased intracompartmental pressure (see p.91).

Contained within the muscle compartment, bruising is unlikely to appear at the surface but sometimes may appear a few days later in a more proximal area. Swelling may not be apparent due to its containment deep inside the muscle, but it can be felt as a hard, dense area, which is painful when palpated. The compartment pressure may prevent muscle contraction for some time, and exercises should not be considered until this has improved.

Intermuscular haematoma Strains can involve more than one muscle or compartment, with the fascia in between also being torn along with the muscle fibres. There will be only a minor increase in pressure in the area, as the effusion of blood will easily disperse into interstitial spaces through the torn fascia. Bruising often appears after 24 hours, sometimes in a more distal area due to gravity. These strains generally recover well and massage during the post-acute stage greatly speeds this up. It is important that the damaged fascia does not heal with the formation of too much scar tissue, as this could restrict the flow of interstitial fluids and impair function.

Chronic injury Chronic muscle problems are often the result of a muscle strain that occurred some time ago (months or even years ago), which was not properly dealt with at the time. Areas of hard, compacted tissue can be felt within the muscle, where the fibres have been bound together with adhesions. These tissues will not function, as they are stuck together and unable to glide freely. Due to the congestion, blood-flow through the area will also be very poor. Over time, the body can get used to this situation and accepts it as 'normal', the sensation of pain diminishes and the healing process stops.

Compartment syndrome Muscles, or compartments within them, can increase in size, due to a rapid increase in strength or through swelling following a trauma. In some situations the fascia surrounding the compartment may not be able to accommodate this increase and will become stretched. Excessive intermuscular pressure will build up, causing pain and impairing function, and will feel hard and painful when palpated. It can also restrict, or even stop, the circulation to distal areas as it compresses blood vessels. In extreme cases it can cause a starvation of blood (necrosis) to distal areas, which is an emergency situation that may require surgery.

Most conditions are quite minor and the commonly affected compartments are in the lower leg. The muscle groups here are contained within a fascia that is naturally quite narrow and tight to maintain their shape. Massage to improve tissue permeability and release tension in the fascial sheath (especially CTM, see Chapter 14), and general techniques to improve circulation work well. Friction should *not* be used in the early stages, as it may cause inflammation, which could increase swelling in the compartment and make the condition worse. Sometimes massage treatment has little effect on this condition, particularly in the deep posterior compartment, and medical treatment may be preferable.

Tendon injuries

Strain (also called a tear or rupture) Most muscles are attached to bones via tendons, which are inelastic and have very strong tensile strength. When the muscle contracts, the force is transmitted through it to create movement at the bone. A tendon is not completely inelastic, because if it were it would not be able to cope with a sudden force. Most tendons can in fact accommodate about a 5 per cent stretch, but a force that causes anything greater than this will result in some fibres tearing.

After the age of about 35, degenerative changes reduce the elasticity of tendons, although sensible regular exercise can delay this. Inflammation will weaken a tendon and also make it more vulnerable to strain. These are important considerations when advising athletes about warm-up programmes, etc.

Tendons are subject to strain if:

- Tension is applied too quickly, especially if not 'warmed-up'.
- The tendon is already tense when force is applied.
- The muscle is maximally contracted when force is applied.
- The muscle is forced into extension by external forces.
- An oblique force is applied.
- The tendon is weak relative to the muscle.

Complete ruptures These are more common in older people who do sports or activities that involve high impact on hard surfaces, such as tennis. The Achilles tendon is most commonly injured in this way.

Symptoms
- The athlete may feel a sudden 'snap' followed by intense pain. (Pain may reduce very quickly, as there is no function to aggravate the tissues.)
- No functional movement is possible, as there is no connection between muscle and bone.
- Swelling and bruising appear quickly.

These injuries are fairly uncommon and a patient will usually go straight to a hospital. Immediate surgical repair is sometimes regarded as the only effective treatment method. Early introduction of massage in post-operative treatment produces good results (see Chapter 17).

Partial ruptures In minor cases a rupture may not be obvious, as the symptoms are much the same as with over-use inflammation. With continued exercise the torn fibres will not repair and excessive scar tissue will build up. This can have considerable long-term consequences, especially in sheathed tendons such as the Achilles. The increased demand placed on the unaffected fibres puts them at risk too. The most commonly affected tendon is the Achilles, but the patella tendon, rotator cuff tendons of the shoulder and adductor longus tendon are other examples.

Acute symptoms
- Sudden onset of pain, usually occurring during a specific event or movement
- Pain occurs if movement is repeated or when the associated joint is moved against resistance.
- Localized pain, swelling and haematoma
- A defect may be felt along the surface of the tendon.

Chronic symptoms
- Although there may be a sudden onset of pain, there may be no obvious cause or trauma.
- Pain may be experienced when warming up; then it eases during moderate exercise, but returns if it becomes more intense.
- Resisted movements at the associated joint may cause pain.
- Localized tenderness and swelling

Acute conditions may require referral as surgical repair is sometimes necessary. In the post-acute or chronic phases, friction massage techniques should be used with caution as they may increase inflammation, especially in sheathed tendons. Application of ice after friction can help prevent this, but sometimes less invasive treatments such as ultrasound may produce better results in the early stages.

Muscle tendon junction A common site for strain and inflammation to occur is at the muscle/tendon junction. These two types of tissue have very different elastic capabilities, and where they merge together shearing forces can occur on a microscopic level. Micro-trauma commonly builds up in this area, and so it should be assessed and treated as a matter of course in any massage treatment, as a preventative measure.

Tendon inflammation (tendinitis) or inflammation of its sheath (peritendonditis, tenovaginitis) A tendon can become inflamed for a variety of reasons.

External factors (examples)
- Heel tabs from shoes rubbing the Achilles tendon
- Tight shoelaces rubbing the tendons in the dorsal foot

Intrinsic factors
- Repetitive movement with a tendon rubbing over a bony prominence, the hip and shoulder being common problem areas. Tight muscles or poor joint alignment (common in the shoulder) can make the tendon pull tighter across the joint and cause it to rub. In sport the problem can also be due to poor technique.
- Rubbing against a ligament or retinaculum, commonly found at the ankle or wrist. Tight muscles in sport, or the repetitive action of the fingers and wrists in typing, could also cause this rubbing effect.
- Repetitive loading from strong or tight muscles causing micro-trauma, the Achilles tendon being the common example.

Some large tendons have a sheath inside, which passes smoothly around a joint. Compression can cause rubbing and inflammation inside this sheath. Scarring inside the sheath can be identified by a creaking sensation (crepitus) when the tendon moves. Scarring outside the sheath will appear as a palpable thickening along the tendon, and this can be effectively broken down using friction techniques. But with scarring inside the sheath, friction could aggravate the condition and possibly cause more inflammation. For this reason it is a good precaution to apply ice after any friction treatment on these tendons.

Nerve problems

Pain and dysfunction affecting parts of the musculoskeletal system could be due to a disruption in the peripheral nerve supply. Although the symptoms may feel as if they originate in the local tissues, the cause of the problem may be referred from somewhere distant along the path of the nerve. There will usually be no sign of any damage in the local tissues, and palpation will not increase or reduce the symptoms very much, if at all. Diffused numbness, tingling or pins and needles are common symptoms associated with nerve disruption.

The entrapment or compression often occurs where a nerve passes round moving joint structures. At peripheral joints, impact trauma, constant pressure or another injury can lead to fibrous scar tissue, which can restrict the free movement of the nerve (tethering). This can lead to referred symptoms, which are usually felt more distally along the limb. Friction techniques may be able to break this scar tissue down and help ease the problem.

Nerve entrapment caused by spinal problems may also result in symptoms being experienced only in a distal area (a neck injury, for example, may only cause numbness in the thumb). Treating the spinal area with massage may have some beneficial effect, but these conditions must be referred for a medical or osteopathic assessment.

13 Specific Muscles

This chapter deals with specific muscles, explaining how they may become injured. There are many other causes of musculoskeletal pain and dysfunction, which are not muscular in origin and where massage may have only a secondary treatment role. Although some of the more common examples of these are included here, it is important for the student to be familiar with the content of the previous chapter before continuing.

Each therapist needs to develop a unique range of working methods that best suits his physical capabilities (strength, weaknesses and flexibility). The treatment methods explained and shown in this chapter are therefore not intended as a comprehensive guide but rather as a set of examples, from which the individual therapist can develop his own particular techniques.

When developing these techniques it is important to be versatile and inventive. Because we study anatomical charts that are two-dimensional, it is easy to fall into the habit of treating the tissues with this same limited view. Tissue injuries rarely occur conveniently on the outer surfaces, so it is important to discover ways of changing the position of the patient and the working position of the therapist. This can make it possible to explore the area as extensively as possible from different directions, angles and depths. Several examples of this are shown here, but the possibilities are endless.

Friction and deep stroking are the main techniques referred to in this chapter because these are the most effective in dealing with scar tissue, fibrous adhesions and muscle tension. But these techniques do not alone produce good results, and must be supported by a considerable amount of general stroking and kneading. These superficial techniques should be used initially to prepare the tissues so that it becomes easier and less painful to work deeper into them. And by loosening and softening the area, any damaged tissues can be identified more clearly. Between short periods of friction these techniques will stimulate the blood-flow through the area, which can help clear away any particles that have been broken down by the friction. Without doing this they may simply re-congest and make the friction a waste of time. So although it is not mentioned repeatedly throughout the text, superficial massage techniques must always be included in this way.

Long-term chronic injuries may result in a complex pattern of tension throughout a large area, due to altered bio-mechanics and compensation factors. It may take a long time to find the specific tissues that are the root cause of the problem. Sometimes the first treatment session may be only a 'softening-up' exercise, with the real work of finding and treating the cause taking place at subsequent sessions.

Soft tissue problems are rarely isolated to just one structure even though it may appear so. Painful symptoms can be referred to distant areas through the nerves or connective tissue. Functionally, a problem in one area can lead to referred symptoms in another, due to compensation. So it is important to explore the tissue in all areas associated with the structure and function of the painful area.

Although chronic problems usually develop deep in the tissues, this is not always the case. It is easy to fall into the habit of working deeper and deeper in an effort to locate areas of damage, but it is occasionally possible to miss a problem in the superficial area by pushing past it. Sometimes light friction is more effective than deep, especially where muscle fascia is involved.

Whenever an area of scar tissue, fibrosis or tension has been treated, it is vitally important to stretch the tissues afterwards to help restore normal length. Although this is mentioned in only a few examples where it is of particular importance, passive stretching should always be applied at the end of any friction treatment.

Reference is made throughout this chapter to treating areas of muscle 'tension' and 'imbalance', which are both only relative terms. The muscles in each individual will have their own normal level of tension (tone), and only where it is excessive or diminished for that individual can it be considered a problem. The difference between the muscle tone of a heavyweight boxer and a ballerina is vast, and to try to reduce tension in the boxer or increase it in the ballerina would be both unnecessary and unwelcome. General relaxation may be another consideration here, as a person who is unable to relax well, or is being affected by other forms of stress (usually psychological), may display high levels of muscle tension regardless of any injury. In this case deep techniques may have little effect initially, and superficial strokes will need to be used much more to aid general relaxation first.

Muscle imbalance is also relative to the individual. Most people are predominantly one-sided (e.g. right-handed), so muscles on one side will become more developed than on the other. Occupational and sporting factors can also create natural imbalances as the musculature develops to meet the repetitive demands. Any noticeable imbalances need to be considered in relation to the way the individual uses his body, and only where it appears to be causing or contributing to an injury, or affecting normal function, should it be considered 'excessive' and in need of specific treatment.

Student's note: Although this chapter contains tables that show the origin, insertion and action of muscles, this is a highly complex subject that has been simplified here for practical reasons. More detailed analysis is available in other specialized texts.

The role of the 'origin' and 'insertion' is one that often reverses. For example, with the levator scapula: the origin is the cervical vertebra when elevating the shoulder, but the scapula insertion becomes the origin when it is fixed and the neck is side-bent. For this reason the *text* mainly refers to them simply as attachments. Also, it should be remembered that people come in a variety of shapes and sizes, and so there will always be slight differences in the exact location of attachments.

The action of individual muscles is an even more complex subject. As the muscular system works as a whole through patterns of movement, it is often difficult to isolate the specific functions of a single component. The tables in this chapter show just the main movements in which a muscle is involved. These are the actions that normally take place through mild contraction from an upright standing position, with the arms down by the sides. When the body is in other positions the pattern of muscular activity changes, as it adapts to cope with the force of gravity coming from a different direction. And, as the force of a particular movement increases, more muscles become involved to stabilize other parts of the body.

1. Back torso
Muscles: superficial and deep

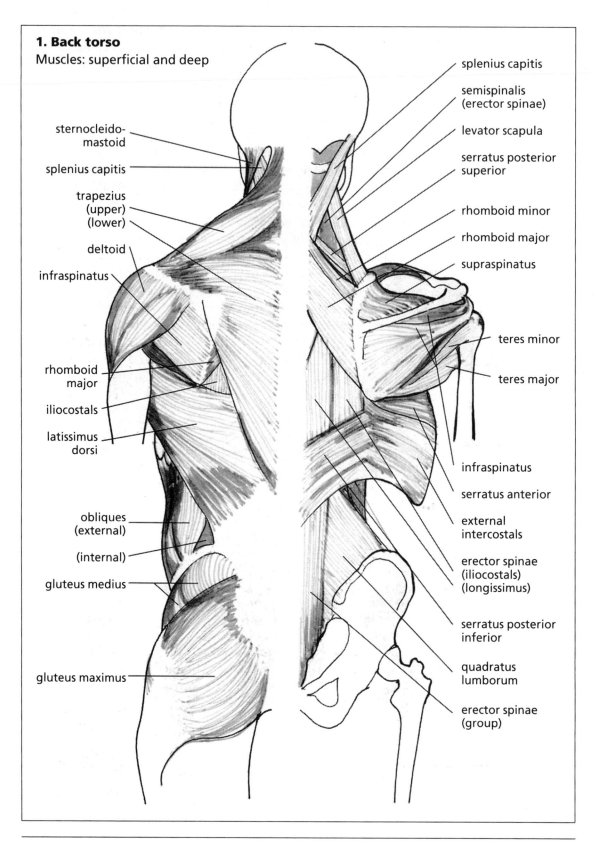

splenius capitis

semispinalis
(erector spinae)

levator scapula

serratus posterior
superior

rhomboid minor

rhomboid major

supraspinatus

teres minor

teres major

infraspinatus

serratus anterior

external
intercostals

erector spinae
(iliocostals)
(longissimus)

serratus posterior
inferior

quadratus
lumborum

erector spinae
(group)

sternocleido-
mastoid

splenius capitis

trapezius
(upper)
(lower)

deltoid

infraspinatus

rhomboid
major

iliocostals

latissimus
dorsi

obliques
(external)

(internal)

gluteus medius

gluteus maximus

2. Back torso Bones and ligaments

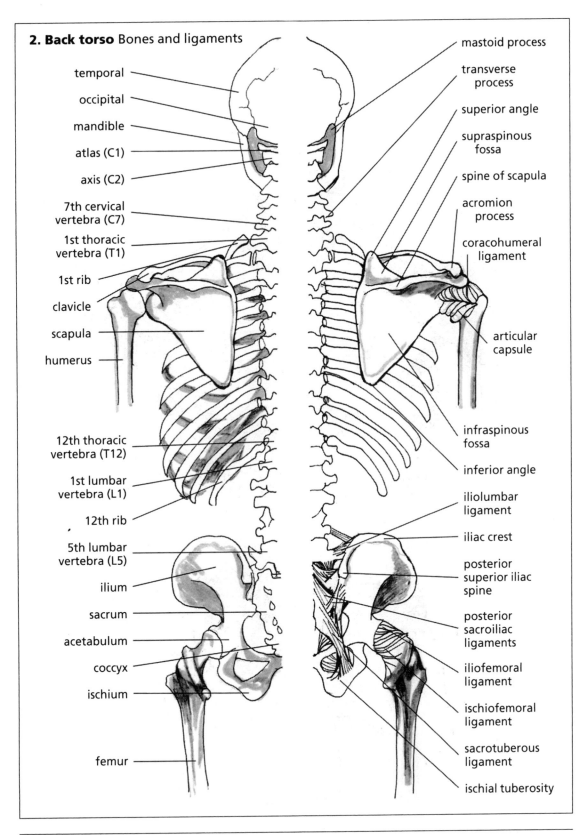

temporal

occipital

mandible

atlas (C1)

axis (C2)

7th cervical
vertebra (C7)

1st thoracic
vertebra (T1)

1st rib

clavicle

scapula

humerus

12th thoracic
vertebra (T12)

1st lumbar
vertebra (L1)

12th rib

5th lumbar
vertebra (L5)

ilium

sacrum

acetabulum

coccyx

ischium

femur

mastoid process

transverse
process

superior angle

supraspinous
fossa

spine of scapula

acromion
process

coracohumeral
ligament

articular
capsule

infraspinous
fossa

inferior angle

iliolumbar
ligament

iliac crest

posterior
superior iliac
spine

posterior
sacroiliac
ligaments

iliofemoral
ligament

ischiofemoral
ligament

sacrotuberous
ligament

ischial tuberosity

3. Front torso
Muscles: superficial and deep

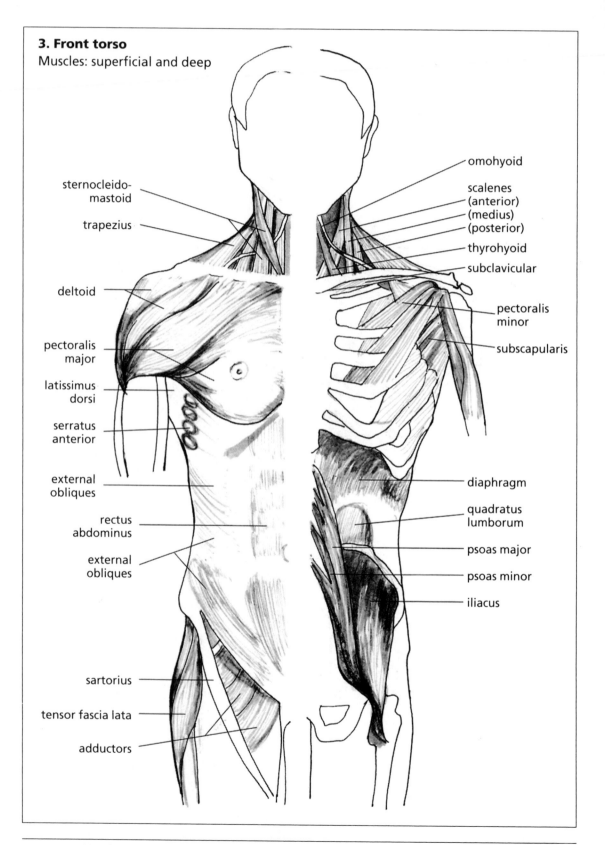

- sternocleido-mastoid
- trapezius
- deltoid
- pectoralis major
- latissimus dorsi
- serratus anterior
- external obliques
- rectus abdominus
- external obliques
- sartorius
- tensor fascia lata
- adductors

- omohyoid
- scalenes (anterior) (medius) (posterior)
- thyrohyoid
- subclavicular
- pectoralis minor
- subscapularis
- diaphragm
- quadratus lumborum
- psoas major
- psoas minor
- iliacus

4. Front torso
Bones and ligaments

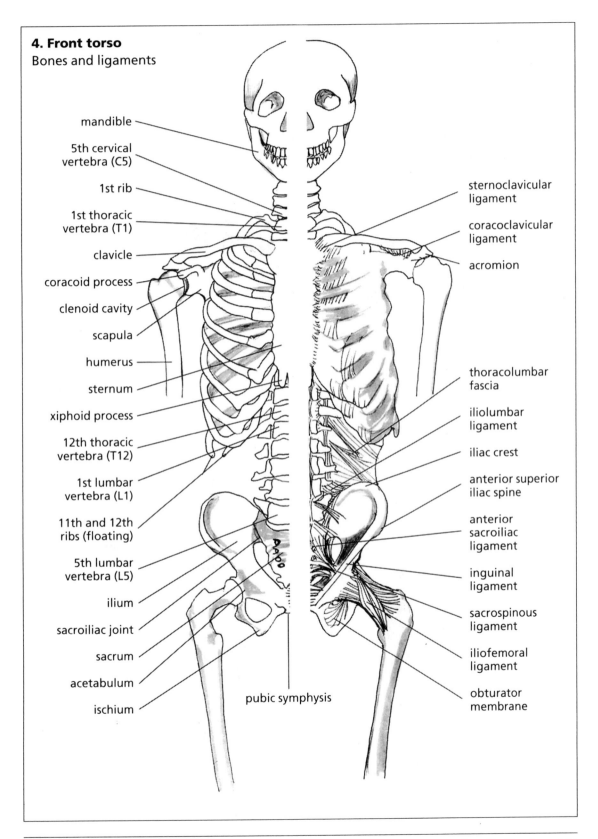

mandible

5th cervical
vertebra (C5)

1st rib

1st thoracic
vertebra (T1)

clavicle

coracoid process

clenoid cavity

scapula

humerus

sternum

xiphoid process

12th thoracic
vertebra (T12)

1st lumbar
vertebra (L1)

11th and 12th
ribs (floating)

5th lumbar
vertebra (L5)

ilium

sacroiliac joint

sacrum

acetabulum

ischium

pubic symphysis

sternoclavicular
ligament

coracoclavicular
ligament

acromion

thoracolumbar
fascia

iliolumbar
ligament

iliac crest

anterior superior
iliac spine

anterior
sacroiliac
ligament

inguinal
ligament

sacrospinous
ligament

iliofemoral
ligament

obturator
membrane

5. Back arm
Muscles: superficial and deep

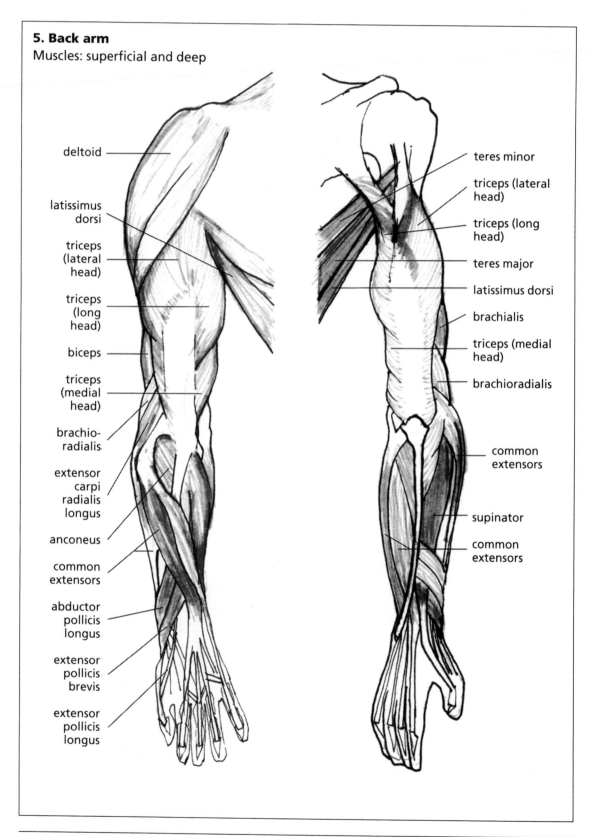

deltoid

latissimus dorsi

triceps (lateral head)

triceps (long head)

biceps

triceps (medial head)

brachio-radialis

extensor carpi radialis longus

anconeus

common extensors

abductor pollicis longus

extensor pollicis brevis

extensor pollicis longus

teres minor

triceps (lateral head)

triceps (long head)

teres major

latissimus dorsi

brachialis

triceps (medial head)

brachioradialis

common extensors

supinator

common extensors

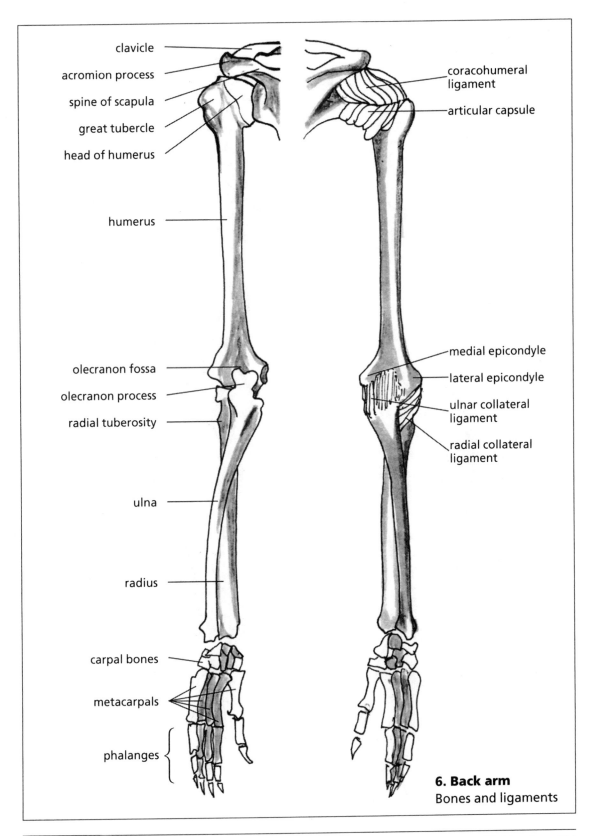

clavicle

acromion process

spine of scapula

great tubercle

head of humerus

humerus

olecranon fossa

olecranon process

radial tuberosity

ulna

radius

carpal bones

metacarpals

phalanges

coracohumeral
ligament

articular capsule

medial epicondyle

lateral epicondyle

ulnar collateral
ligament

radial collateral
ligament

6. Back arm
Bones and ligaments

7. Front arm
Muscles: superficial and deep

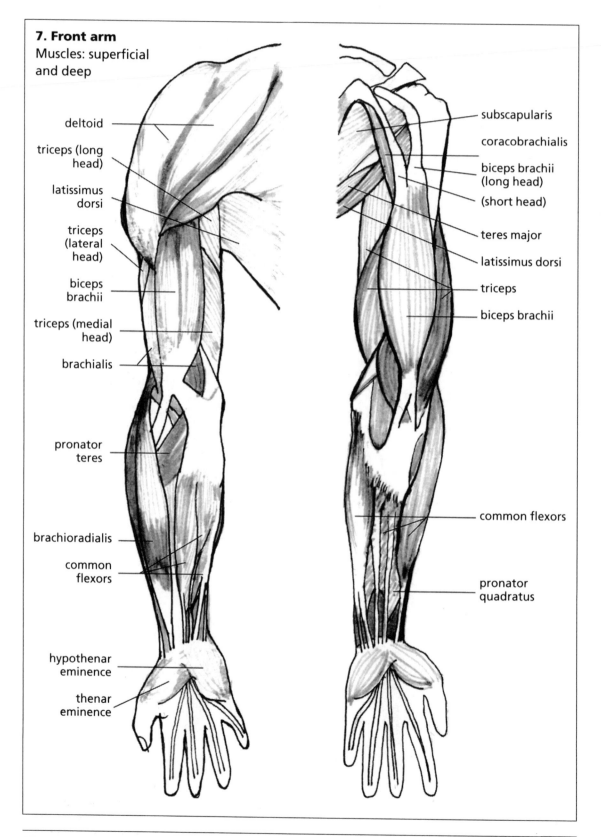

deltoid

triceps (long head)

latissimus dorsi

triceps (lateral head)

biceps brachii

triceps (medial head)

brachialis

pronator teres

brachioradialis

common flexors

hypothenar eminence

thenar eminence

subscapularis

coracobrachialis

biceps brachii (long head)

(short head)

teres major

latissimus dorsi

triceps

biceps brachii

common flexors

pronator quadratus

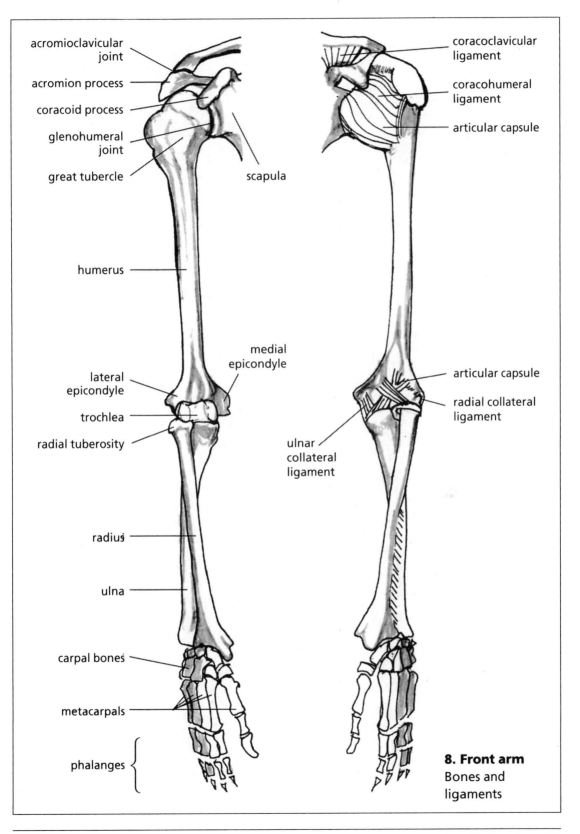

acromioclavicular joint

acromion process

coracoid process

glenohumeral joint

great tubercle

scapula

humerus

medial epicondyle

lateral epicondyle

trochlea

radial tuberosity

radius

ulna

carpal bones

metacarpals

phalanges

coracoclavicular ligament

coracohumeral ligament

articular capsule

articular capsule

radial collateral ligament

ulnar collateral ligament

8. Front arm
Bones and ligaments

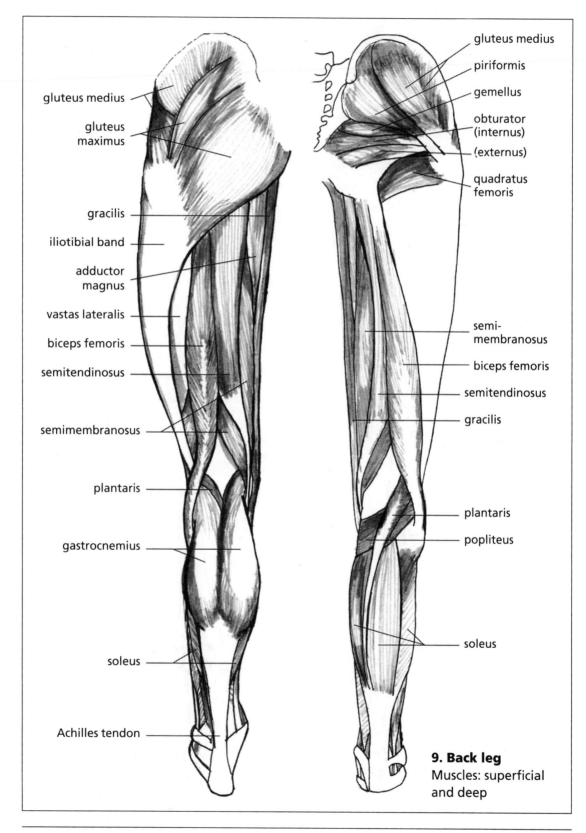

gluteus medius

gluteus
maximus

gracilis

iliotibial band

adductor
magnus

vastas lateralis

biceps femoris

semitendinosus

semimembranosus

plantaris

gastrocnemius

soleus

Achilles tendon

gluteus medius

piriformis

gemellus

obturator
(internus)

(externus)

quadratus
femoris

semi-
membranosus

biceps femoris

semitendinosus

gracilis

plantaris

popliteus

soleus

9. Back leg
Muscles: superficial
and deep

10. Back leg
Bones and ligaments

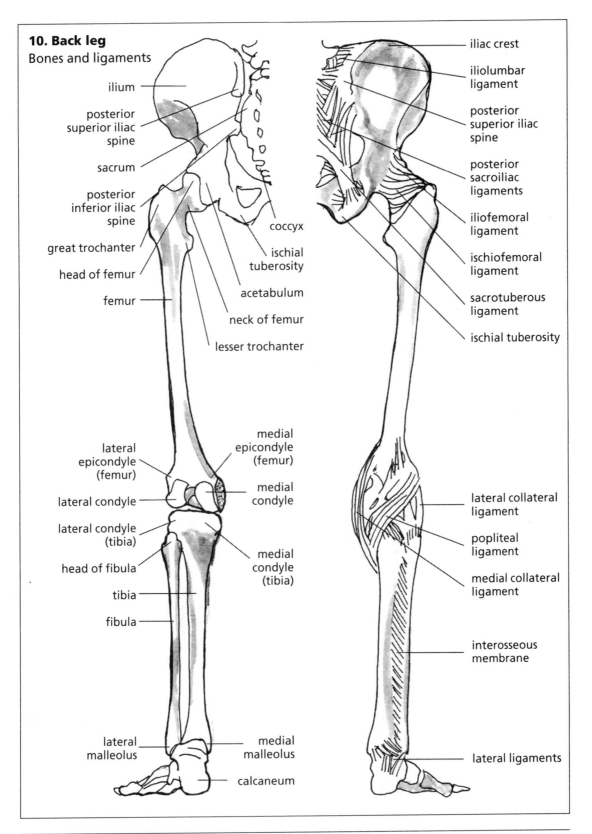

ilium

posterior superior iliac spine

sacrum

posterior inferior iliac spine

great trochanter

head of femur

femur

coccyx

ischial tuberosity

acetabulum

neck of femur

lesser trochanter

lateral epicondyle (femur)

lateral condyle

lateral condyle (tibia)

head of fibula

tibia

fibula

medial epicondyle (femur)

medial condyle

medial condyle (tibia)

lateral malleolus

medial malleolus

calcaneum

iliac crest

iliolumbar ligament

posterior superior iliac spine

posterior sacroiliac ligaments

iliofemoral ligament

ischiofemoral ligament

sacrotuberous ligament

ischial tuberosity

lateral collateral ligament

popliteal ligament

medial collateral ligament

interosseous membrane

lateral ligaments

11. Front leg
Muscles: superficial and deep

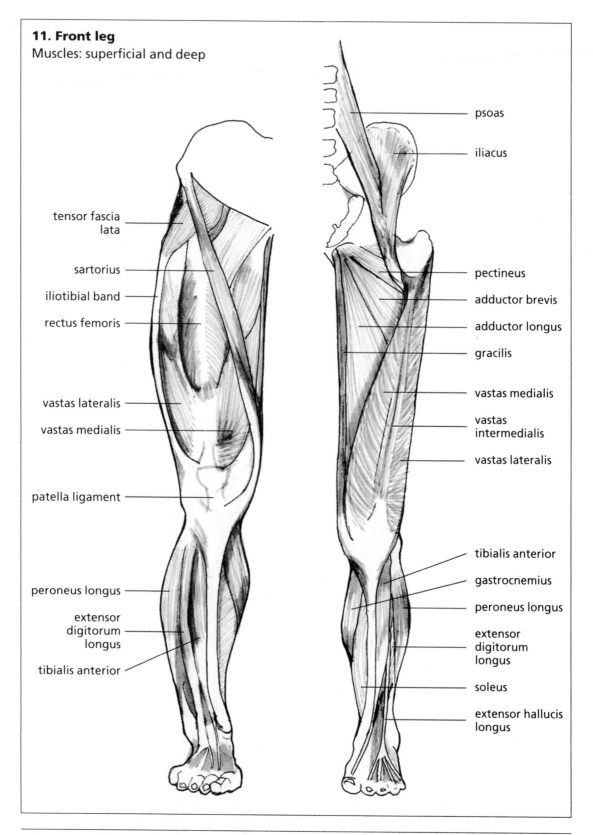

tensor fascia lata

sartorius

iliotibial band

rectus femoris

vastas lateralis

vastas medialis

patella ligament

peroneus longus

extensor digitorum longus

tibialis anterior

psoas

iliacus

pectineus

adductor brevis

adductor longus

gracilis

vastas medialis

vastas intermedialis

vastas lateralis

tibialis anterior

gastrocnemius

peroneus longus

extensor digitorum longus

soleus

extensor hallucis longus

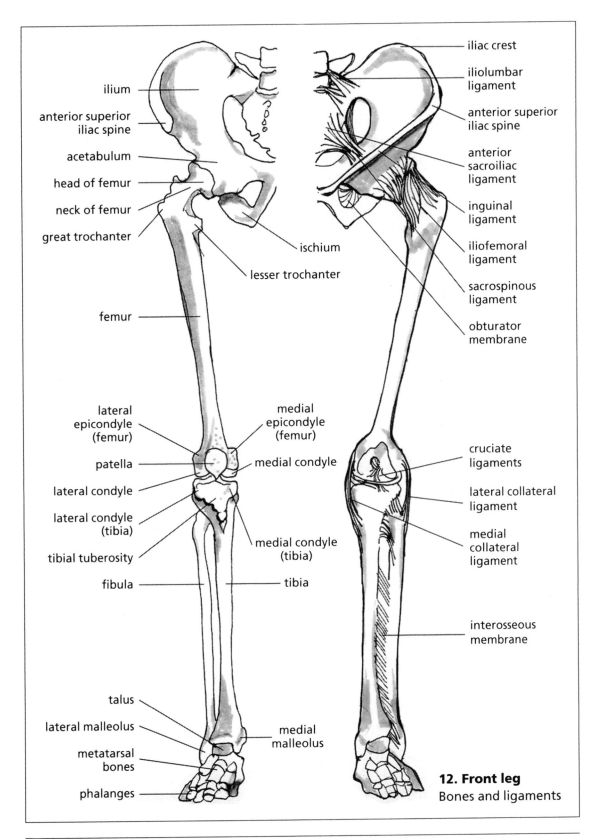

ilium

anterior superior
iliac spine

acetabulum

head of femur

neck of femur

great trochanter

ischium

lesser trochanter

femur

iliac crest

iliolumbar
ligament

anterior superior
iliac spine

anterior
sacroiliac
ligament

inguinal
ligament

iliofemoral
ligament

sacrospinous
ligament

obturator
membrane

lateral
epicondyle
(femur)

medial
epicondyle
(femur)

patella

medial condyle

lateral condyle

lateral condyle
(tibia)

medial condyle
(tibia)

tibial tuberosity

fibula

tibia

cruciate
ligaments

lateral collateral
ligament

medial
collateral
ligament

interosseous
membrane

talus

lateral malleolus

metatarsal
bones

phalanges

medial
malleolus

12. Front leg
Bones and ligaments

Torso and neck

Student's note: THE SPINE

The adult spine is made up of 26 bones and is described in sections, according to their size and curvature. From the top:

- *7 cervical vertebrae (C1 to C7) are quite small and have a natural lordotic curve. Atlas and axis (C1, C2) at the top are structurally different from the rest and form a pivot joint.*
- *12 thoracic vertebrae (T1 to T12), sometimes called dorsal (D1 to D12), are a little larger and have a natural kyphotic curve. The ribs attach to them.*
- *5 lumbar vertebrae (L1 to L5) are the largest and take the greatest weight-bearing load. They have a natural lordotic curve.*
- *The sacrum bone is made up of 5 bones (S1 to S5), which fuse together during puberty. It attaches to the iliac bone, forming a major weight-bearing joint (sacroiliac).*
- *The coccyx comprises 4 bones that also fuse together at the base of the spine and form the only part of the spine that is not weight-bearing.*

There are 24 discs between the vertebrae, which make up one-third of the overall length of the spine. These discs, along with the natural curvatures, absorb impact and enable the spine to cope with weight-bearing situations.

Erector spinae and deep spinal muscles

MUSCLE	ORIGIN	INSERTION	ACTION
Iliocostals	Sacrum, iliac crest and ribs	Ribs and cervical vertebrae	Bilaterally: extends spine
Longissimus	Sacrum, lower thoracic and lumbar vertebrae	Cervical and lower thoracic vertebrae, and mastoid process	Unilaterally: side-bends spine
Spinalis			Extends and rotates head
Interspinalis	Connects transverse and spinous processes		All intervertebral movements
Multifidis			
Semispinalis			

The erector spinae and deep spinal muscles form a complex network of muscles that bind the spinal column together.

The more superficial muscles run along the spine, connecting adjacent bones or spanning several bones along the whole structure. These enable extension to occur, with a degree of independence in each vertebra and each spinal section. The more lateral muscles connect to the ribs, which makes them closely involved in breathing as well as assisting in side-bending. The deep muscles run obliquely between different spinous processes on adjacent vertebrae and these enable a degree of independent rotation between them. As well as initiating movement, they also have an important stabilizing function when other parts of the body, or segments of the spine, are moving.

Acute strains are common in heavy lifting activities, and poor technique or co-ordination is often a contributory factor. If a powerful lift is attempted by moving only one part of the back, the muscles in that section can become strained. Where tension and restricted function exist in one section of the spine, the sections above and/or below it will tend to compensate and also become more prone to injury. For this reason it is important to treat the whole of the spine thoroughly and not just the sections where painful symptoms appear.

Structural injuries to the vertebrae or discs will cause a degree of protective spasm within this muscle group. Back pain and dysfunction may appear to come from the muscles only, but structural problems should always be considered. Although very rare, in extreme cases it is possible that the protective spasm may actually hold damaged structure in place, and by releasing the spasm with massage the bones may become displaced and symptoms could suddenly become much worse.

There is also a very complex network of ligaments linking all the vertebrae together, and if these are injured they will also cause local muscle spasm. Injuries caused by an overload within the normal range of movement will normally only affect the muscles. But if an extreme range of movement is involved, as perhaps occurs in a fall, damage to the ligaments is more likely. With an overload in an extreme range, the disc or vertebra becomes more vulnerable to injury. Bilateral muscle spasm can be the symptom of structural damage, whereas a muscle injury is more likely to be unilateral.

Most back movements involve some action or control from all the vertebrae, so even a very small area of damage, which may only directly affect a single joint, can cause considerable pain and dysfunction over a large area. Patients sometimes have extremely dramatic symptoms but apart from general muscular spasm it may be difficult to find the actual site of damage, which could be no thicker than a human hair.

The erector spinae muscles commonly suffer from over-use tension due to postural, occupational or repetitive stress. Chronic muscular imbalances can lead to further postural problems elsewhere. Rarely will the whole group be affected in the same way, and excessive tension can be found in one area, with weakness in another. Tension on one side of the spine will inhibit and cause weakness to muscles on the other. So a pattern of tension and weakness can develop all the way along both sides of the spine. As tension draws some joints together and weakness allows others to be drawn apart, excessive curvatures and rotations can develop and become permanent after a time. If there is a curvature in one segment of the spine, the next segment will develop the opposite curvature in an effort to keep the trunk upright and the eyes level.

The common areas for tension are:

- Cervical area, due to the muscles shortening because of increased curvature of the vertebrae
- Mid-thoracic area, as many of the muscles coming from both above and below attach here, making it subject to stress from opposite directions
- Lumbar area, due to muscle shortening for many reasons, particularly a forward-tilting pelvis and weak abdominal muscles. The lower back can also suffer from constant compression during running or jumping activities, especially with a tilted pelvis and weak abdominals.

Long strokes can be applied down the erector spinae muscles to help straighten an excessive thoracic curvature.

Treatment

Treating the erector spinae is a major part of any back massage treatment. Before starting, the therapist should observe the patient's posture (standing, sitting and moving) to assess the areas of tension and restriction. The patient should then lie in a comfortable prone position on the couch, using cushions – usually under the hips and/or shoulders – to achieve the best relaxation.

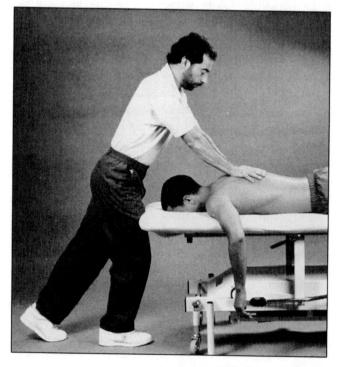

Long strokes can be performed both up the back and down it. If the patient has excessive curvature in the thoracic spine (kyphosis), strokes down this section of the spine will encourage the feeling of a straighter back and also provide a better position from which to apply deep pressure. With excessive curvature in the lumbar area (lordosis), short strokes down towards the sacrum work well for the same reasons. Otherwise, strokes should generally go up the back. Deep, long strokes can be applied along the spine, using both thumbs on either side of the spinous processes. This is a good way of identifying the segments or vertebrae that are particularly tense, congested or possibly out of alignment.

To identify tight or damaged muscle bands within the group, deep transverse stokes are the most effective. The therapist should stand on

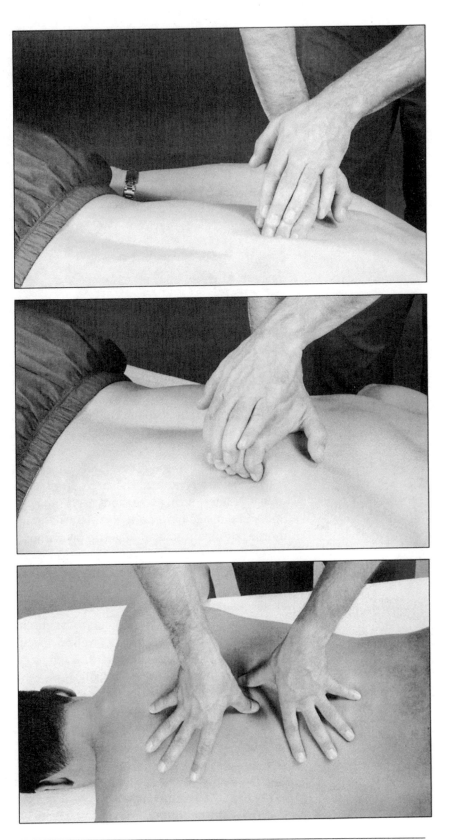

Friction with the fingertips (pushing) into the lateral fibres of the erector spinae muscles.

Using the fingers in a hooked position, friction can be applied deeply beneath the lateral fibres of the erector spinae muscles (pulling).

Friction can be applied with the thumbs into the deep muscles and ligaments around the spine.

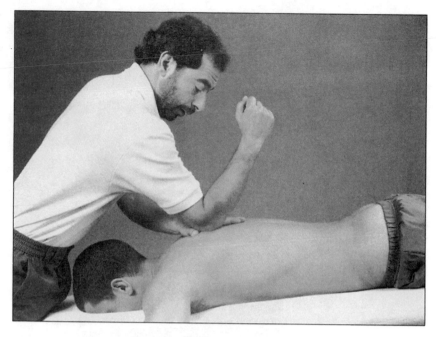

Deep friction can be applied with the elbow into the deep muscles and ligaments around the spine.

one side of the couch to apply lateral strokes to the muscles on the opposite side of the spine. The thumb or fingers should apply a deep downward pressure next to the spinous processes and then a stroke can be pushed laterally through the muscles. It can also be applied in the other direction by curling the fingers into the lateral fibres and pulling back.

As there are so many layers of muscle, it takes time to be able to reach the deepest tissues. These stroking techniques should be returned to many times during a session, each time exploring deeper layers. To find any damage close to the spine usually necessitates very deep and thorough palpation, with fingertip precision.

Once located, these areas of tension or scarring should be treated with deep friction. This can cause considerable pain and the NMT principles (see Chapter 14) can be used to good effect. One key area to treat in this way is around the lower lumbar and sacral attachments, where important ligaments, in particular the iliolumbar ligament, are also located. Fibrosis and tension as well as specific areas of tissue damage are common here, and can lead to referred problems elsewhere in the back or hip. As well as mechanically dealing with these situations, very deep pressure has a strong neuromuscular effect, which can release tension over a wide area.

The lateral border of the muscle group often requires particular attention, especially in the lumbar area. If the oblique abdominal muscles are weak, the lateral fibres become more involved in side-bending and can therefore suffer from over-use. This can be treated with friction in towards the spinous processes, with the patient in a side-lying position (with the quadratus lumborum, see p.117).

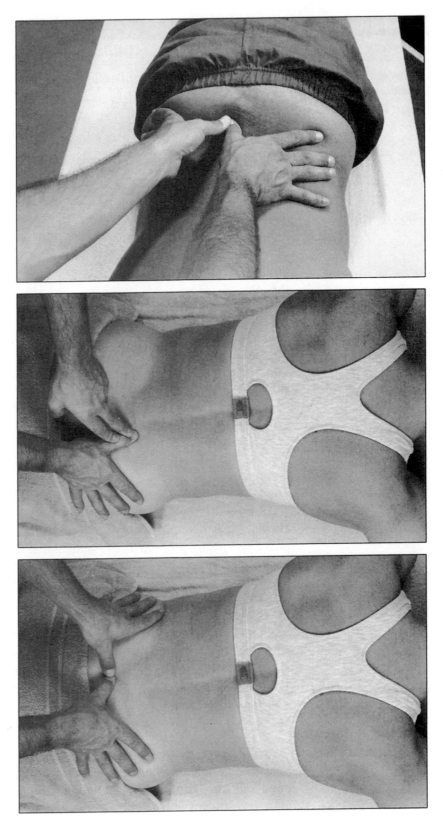

Deep friction with the thumbs down into the iliolumbar ligament.

Deep transverse strokes with the thumb into the erector spinae insertion and iliolumbar ligament.

Friction applied with the thumbs around the sacroiliac joint.

Quadratus lumborum (QL)

MUSCLE	ORIGIN	INSERTION	ACTION
Quadratus lumborum	Iliac crest	12th rib, L1 to L4/5	Bilaterally: extends lower back Unilaterally: side-bends trunk

This is a very deep muscle, much of which lies beneath the erector spinae. As well as being a main lateral flexor and assisting back extension, bilaterally it is the major stabilizer of the lumbar pelvic area and is therefore vitally important when lifting and holding heavy objects. The muscle also plays a secondary role in abduction of the hip by raising the ilium, and as it also attaches to the bottom rib it is involved in breathing, too.

Acute strains often occur in heavy lifting activities, especially if other trunk movements are also involved. These can cause considerable muscle spasm, severe dysfunction and sometimes even a postural distortion. Chronic tension can develop through repetitive use and other postural problems can also lead to imbalances between the two sides.

Both QL muscles and both iliopsoas muscles (see p.186) reciprocally oppose one another, and any imbalances should be considered between all *four*.

Treatment

The QL is a difficult muscle to treat because it is mostly hidden by the erector spinae when the patient is lying straight in the prone position. Having the patient curve his trunk over to one side, in a 'banana'-like position, opens up the area and pulls the erector spinae towards the centre. This makes the lateral fibres, which are more prone to injury, more accessible. In this position deep friction can be applied from the iliac crest along to the lower rib.

To reach the medial fibres, where chronic tension is more likely, friction needs to be directed from the lateral border in towards the spine. The erector spinae muscles must be softened and relaxed first as much as possible to allow the fingers to get in between the two muscles. These frictions are best applied with the patient in the side-lying position, with the area opened up by the patient abducting the (upper) arm and straightening the (upper) leg.

Lumbar fascia Extending superficially over the lower back is a thick fascia, which binds the muscles together and serves as the origin for the latissimus dorsi and some of the oblique abdominal muscles. It is treated along with the other lower back muscles.

With the patient lying in a curved position with his arm abducted, the lateral fibres of the quadratus lumborum can be reached. Friction can be applied with the fingers in a hooked position being pulled medially into the muscle.

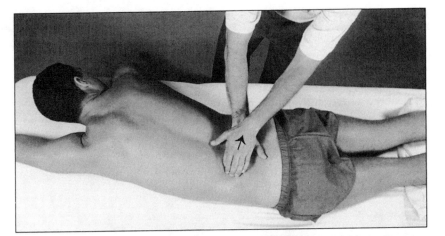

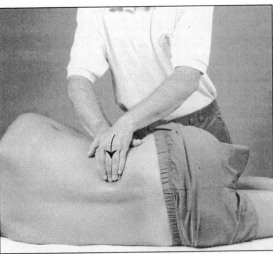

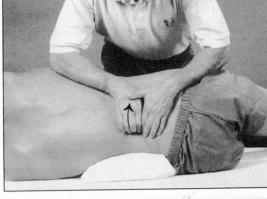

Above (left): With the patient in a side-lying position, the therapist can work down into the lateral fibres and apply friction between the quadratus lumborum and underlying erector spinae muscles.
Above (right): With hooked fingers, the therapist can pull up into the lateral fibres.

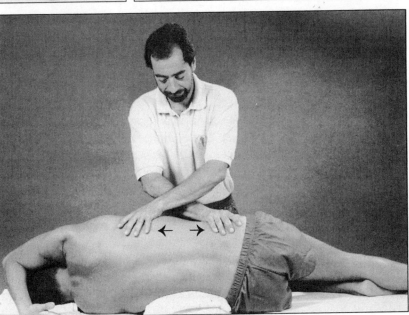

In a side-lying position, bilateral strokes can be applied to stretch the quadratus lumborum.

Posterior neck muscles			
MUSCLE	ORIGIN	INSERTION	ACTION
Splenius capitis	C7 to T3/4	Mastoid process, occiput, transverse process of atlas	Extends and rotates head
Splenius cervicis	T4 to T6		
Semispinalis	C3/4 to T5	Occiput	
Capitis	Transverse and spinous processes of atlas and axis		

This is a complex group of muscles, which runs up the back of the neck, and all are involved in extension and rotation of the head and neck.

Due to the weight of the head, these muscles are under constant tension when in an upright position. Holding the head in a fixed position (isometric contraction), such as when leaning over a desk or riding a bike, can increase tension in the particular muscles that are under the greatest strain.

Postural imbalances in the neck and shoulders will also affect the muscles, the most common being a shortening due to increased curvature in the cervical vertebrae. A postural neck problem should not be seen in isolation, as it may be a symptom of imbalances lower down the body. For example, if the upper chest area is tight, the shoulders and upper thoracic spine get pulled forward and the cervical spine then has to increase its curvature, by muscle contraction, to maintain the head in the upright position.

Acute injuries are common in falls or accidents, due to the sudden extreme force on the muscles to prevent rapid movement of the head (whiplash). Almost everyone who lives an active (or inactive) life will suffer at some time from this type of injury. Considerable protective spasm will occur with an acute injury to prevent neck movement during initial recovery, and symptoms may appear quite dramatic even when there is only a small amount of tissue damage.

After acute injuries the tissues often do not fully recover their normal length, because it is too easy to compensate for restricted movement by using the shoulders and trunk more. Chronic tension can often develop unnoticed for the same reason. In the long term this could lead to painful symptoms in other areas, but treating these without dealing properly with the neck will achieve very little.

A common area of tension is in the nape of the neck, just below the occipital bone. This is because in a forward-leaning position the deep muscles, particularly the capitis and splenii, are under constant isometric contraction as they hold the head up. Tightness and congestion here can restrict circulation of the blood and cerebrospinal fluid and affect nerve stimulation to the head, and this is one of the most common causes of headaches.

Treatment

As there are so many muscles in this area it needs to be assessed very thoroughly. In most people there is usually some tension in certain muscles, due to past injury, and even though they may cause little pain when palpated, they still require treatment as they could be contributing to other problems. Congestion can also build up around cervical joints and ligaments due to restricted movement. Friction here can release the joint and promote better function in all the tissues.

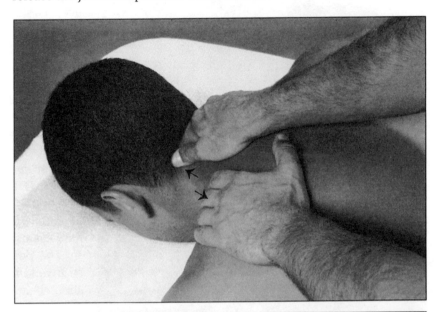

Long strokes can be applied up and/or down the neck muscles.

Deep friction with the fingertips into the sub-occipital region.

Deep friction with the thumb into the deep muscles and ligaments around the cervical vertebrae.

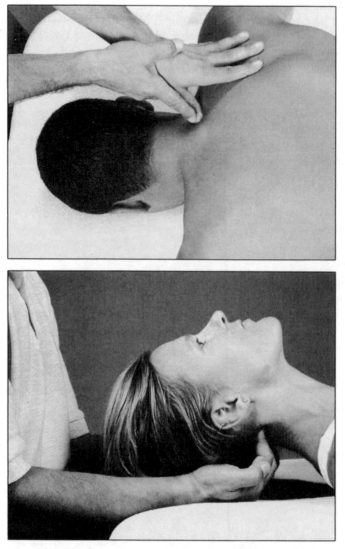

In the prone position, transverse stoking can be used to identify tight or damaged muscle bands, which can then be treated with friction. Longitudinal strokes can be applied both up and down the area. To work up the muscles, the therapist should stand to the side of the couch and use one hand to fix the shoulder down. Then the thumb, fingers or heel of the other hand can be used to stroke up to the occiput and stretch the muscle. Downward strokes are done from the head, using one hand to pull gently and hold the base of the skull so that the neck is slightly stretched out. The other hand is then used to stroke down the neck muscles.

Friction into the deep tissues beneath the occiput (in the nape of the neck) can be done with the therapist standing at the head or side of the couch, and both positions can be used to work the area thoroughly. This can produce considerable pain and NMT principles (see Chapter 14) should be used, and care should be taken not to squash the tissues hard against the bone.

The posterior muscles can also be treated in the supine position to good effect. Standing at the head of the couch, the therapist can reach with his hands under the patient's neck, and by leaning back, through straight arms, he can apply deep strokes into the tissues in both longitudinal and transverse directions. It is sometimes difficult for the patient to relax into this technique, so the strokes should be made

Stroking and friction techniques can be applied with the patient in the supine position. The therapist curls his fingers up into the tissues and the pressure comes from the weight of the patient's head.

slowly and the pressure gradually increased. At the top of the long stroke the fingers can reach deeply into the sub-occipital area, where friction and NMT can be applied. This is also an excellent position in which to apply a passive stretch by gently pulling the base of the occipital bone.

The levator scapula and upper trapezius overlie the posterior neck muscles, but as they are primarily considered shoulder muscles they are dealt with later (see pp.131 and 129). In practical terms, however, they are treated along with these neck muscles.

Lateral and anterior neck muscles

MUSCLE	ORIGIN	INSERTION	ACTION
Scalene(s): anterior, medius, posterior	C2 to C7	1st and 2nd rib (lateral)	Side-bends and rotates head Raises ribs (inspiration)
Sternocleidomastoid	Sternum and clavicle	Mastoid process	Flexes, rotates and side-bends head

The *scalene* muscles run down the sides of the neck and are primarily used in side-bending the head and neck, but also assist in rotation. Attaching to the upper ribs, they are accessory breathing muscles. Postural misalignment in the cervical spine and also in the jaw will affect the balance between the muscles on the two sides.

Acute injury can occur with sudden or forced side-bending. Tension can build up through over-use in predominantly one-sided sports, or activities such as carrying a shoulder bag or prolonged use of the telephone, all due to sustained isometric contraction. Pain from these muscles is often felt more in the back of the neck. It can also cause referred pain down the patient's arm, because tension or injury to the scalenes can impinge on the brachial nerve plexus, which runs through it.

The *sternocleidomastoid* muscles can usually be seen standing out slightly on either side of the front of the neck, and form the main rotator and flexor muscles of the head.

They can suffer acute injury due to sudden or forced rotation movements of the head. They can become tense and shorten when postural imbalances cause the head to stay in a forward position. Chronic conditions may not cause pain locally because the patient will simply hold the muscle in a shortened position so as not to feel it. This can lead to neck and shoulder problems developing elsewhere, so these muscles should always be treated in association with all other neck and shoulder problems.

Treatment

To treat these muscles in the prone position, the patient's head should be rotated and/or side-bent to enable better access. To do this the therapist should place his whole hand around the base of the skull, almost reaching the ear on the other side. By flexing his wrist, the head will roll in to rest on the forearm.

The therapist should also try to place his abdomen against the crown of the patient's head (the patient may need to move up the couch to enable this to be done). In this position the head and neck can be adjusted, with good support, control and comfort, by the therapist moving his body.

With the head supported
in a slightly side-bent and
rotated position, the
therapist can use the
thumb of his other hand
to stroke and lightly
friction the scalene
muscles.

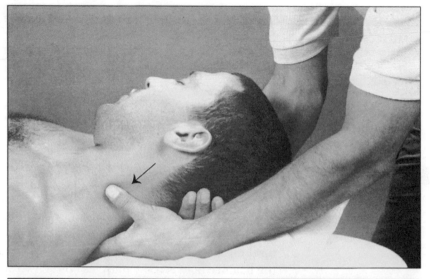

Friction with the fingertip
into the muscle origins
around the mastoid
process.

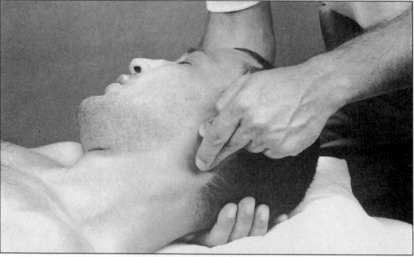

In the supine position,
with the head rotated in
order to treat the
sternocleidomastoid.
Stroking or friction
techniques can be applied
using a pinching action
between the thumb and
fingers. This prevents any
possible damage to the
underlying blood vessels.

Deep stroking along the scalenes down towards the lateral part of the top ribs can release tension locally and throughout the neck area. But friction should not be used too deeply, as this could compress the carotid artery and jugular vein, which lie beneath these muscles.

The sternocleidomastoid is also difficult to treat with deep techniques as, being so close to the throat, it can be irritating and cause the patient to cough; and it may also compress underlying blood vessels. Deep stroking and friction can be achieved by grasping or pinching across the whole muscle and then lifting it away from the underlying structures. In this position a friction can be applied between the therapist's thumb and fingers.

The holding position for the head, described on p.121, should be used for passively stretching the neck muscles. The head and neck can be moved through all ranges of flexion, rotation and side-bending to isolate and stretch specific muscles. MET techniques (see Chapter 14) should be applied to this position also.

Abdominal wall

MUSCLE	ORIGIN	INSERTION	ACTION
External obliques	Lateral surface of 5th to 12th ribs	Abdominal aponeurosis and lower 3 ribs	Rotates, flexes and side-bends trunk
Internal obliques	Iliac crest and lumbar fascia		Supports viscera and assists forced exhalation
Transverse obliques	7th to 12th ribs, lumbar fascia and iliac crest		
Rectus abdominus	Pubis	Costal cartilage, 5th to 7th ribs and base of sternum	Flexes trunk

The oblique muscles wrap around the trunk to the front and centre of the abdomen. The fibres run diagonally down towards the centre (external), up to the centre (internal) and medially (transverse). As well as flexing and rotating the trunk, they assist the diaphragm in forced exhalation.

The rectus abdomini are the long, powerful muscles running down the front of the abdomen which, by connecting the pubis to the ribcage, are central in maintaining a good upright posture. These are the main trunk flexors, and the lower part is also involved in assisting hip flexion. With the obliques, they also support the viscera.

Acute injury is not common in these muscles, but hard, unaccustomed exercise can lead to minor strain. Recovery is usually very quick,

To treat the abdominal muscles with deep techniques they need to be slightly contracted, by the patient actively raising his head. Friction can be applied with the fingertips wherever necessary.

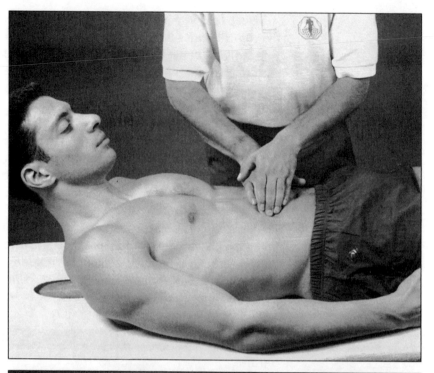

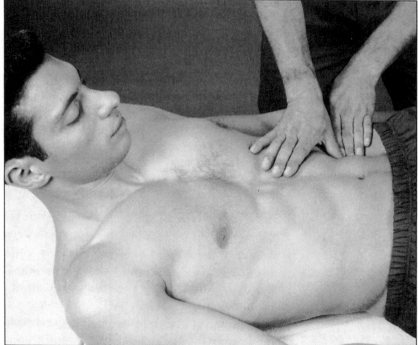

Friction can be applied deeply into the lateral fibres of the rectus abdominus using the thumb and fingers.

due to the rich blood supply and also because the area is easy to rest. The powerful rectus abdomini attach at a very small area, the pubis, which may not be able to cope with the force of contraction, and acute strain can occur here (groin strain).

The muscles are more likely to weaken and stretch, due to poor posture, than to tighten. Chronic tension can also develop in association with medical conditions affecting the abdomen. The link between emotional stress and the condition of the muscles is frequently seen most strongly in the abdomen, where it often seems to increase tension. If this becomes chronic, over a long period it can lead to visceral problems. Tension and painful trigger-points can also form in the abdomen as a result of strong protective muscle spasm to protect a lower back injury.

Abdominal pain could be due to a muscle problem or to a visceral one, and the history of the pain usually gives some indication as to the cause. Any local area of discomfort should be pressed gently to cause a slight pain. Then the patient should contract the muscles by attempting to raise the head and shoulders (knees elevated to protect the lower back). As the only change to take place is in the muscle, if the pain increases, then the problem is more likely to be a muscular one. If there is any doubt whether there may be a visceral organ involved, the patient should be referred to their doctor.

Student's note: When bending forward in a standing position, although the trunk flexes, the abdominal muscles play no part in this. Gravity provides the force, with the back and hip extensors eccentrically contracting to control the movement.

Treatment

It is difficult to apply any deep massage techniques, because the muscles will only sink into the soft viscera beneath. Squeezing and petrissage are the main techniques used, and slightly deeper stroking and friction will have some effect on any specific area of tension. Tissue damage near the pubis attachment, which is usually associated with groin strain, can be treated with deep friction to very good effect, but due to its proximity to the genital area great care and professionalism are needed.

If the muscles are well-toned and with good definition, it is possible to feel the lateral borders of the rectus abdominus. Friction can be applied from here transversely between the muscles. It is sometimes possible to place the fingers round one lateral border and the thumbs along the other, then both muscles can be grasped and lifted away from the underlying tissues. These techniques can help release any tension and adhesions with the muscle attachments to the abdominal aponeurosis.

Abdominal aponeurosis This is a flat sheet of strong, tendinous fibres that runs from the xiphoid process at the base of the sternum to the pubic symphysis. Its lateral borders provide the attachments for some of the oblique muscles. It is treated along with the rectus abdominus.

Respiratory muscles

Diaphragm			
MUSCLE	ORIGIN	INSERTION	ACTION
Diaphragm	Sternum, costal cartilage and 7th to 12th ribs, upper 2/3 lumbar vertebrae	Central tendon	Inhalation

The diaphragm is the most important respiratory muscle. It is a large sheet of muscle, which separates the thoracic and abdominal cavities. The fibres originate from the bottom ribs and lumbar spine, and converge into a strong central tendon. In its resting position it is upwardly domed, and when it contracts it is drawn downwards into the abdomen and a vacuum is created in the chest cavity. The vacuum is filled by air, which is sucked into the lungs. As the muscle relaxes, the diaphragm returns to its domed position and gently pushes the air out of the lungs. The muscle contraction produces inhalation but exhalation is achieved only through its relaxation.

When respiratory demands are slightly higher, during moderate exercise, the diaphragm contracts more quickly and with more force to increase the oxygen intake. But it cannot actively increase exhalation, so instead the oblique muscles contract to increase abdominal pressure. This pushes the diaphragm up with greater force, which clears the lungs quickly and more effectively.

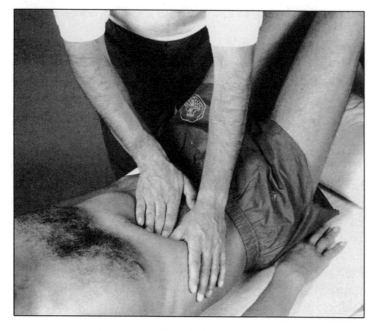

The anterior fibres of the diaphragm can be reached by slowly working the thumb or fingers under the bottom ribs.

Treatment

It is possible to reach the anterior part of the diaphragm with pressure and friction techniques. First the abdomen needs to be treated to soften and relax it. The patient must be supported with cushions so that the neck and upper back, and also the knees, are well elevated. In this position the therapist can work the thumb or fingers up behind the front of the lower ribs to the anterior attachments of the muscle. Although it is not possible to treat the bulk of it directly, this technique can have a strong neuromuscular effect on the whole muscle.

Intercostal muscles

MUSCLE	ORIGIN	INSERTION	ACTION
Internal intercostal	Cross between adjacent ribs		Exhalation
External intercostal			Inhalation

There are two layers of intercostal muscles, which run in a criss-cross pattern between the ribs. The intricate pattern of the fibres can draw the ribs both together and apart and so assist inhalation and exhalation.

The lower intercostals often get injured in impact situations, which in the acute stage can make breathing very painful. If the tissues remain tight and adhered there can be a permanent restriction in lung capacity, which in the case of an athlete may be highly significant. Chronic tension can also develop in association with respiratory conditions (see Chapter 17).

Treatment

The intercostals can be treated with long, deep stroking and friction applied between the ribs, usually with the tips of the fingers. The lower muscles can be covered all the way from the spine to the sternum using supine, side-lying and prone positions, but higher up it is necessary to try to work through the overlying muscles in the front and under the scapula at the back.

Below (left): A stroking technique with the fingertip along the lateral and anterior part of three intercostal muscles at the same time.

Below (right): Deep friction with the fingertips into the intercostal muscle.

Direct treatment to the intercostals under the breast is not possible. However deep friction, using NMT principles (see Chapter 14), at the sternocostal joints can release tension all the way along the muscle. When treating women it is better to work through a towel to give the patient a greater feeling of security. By taking care to work accurately just with the fingertips along the border of the sternum, this becomes a very effective and acceptable technique (see p.128).

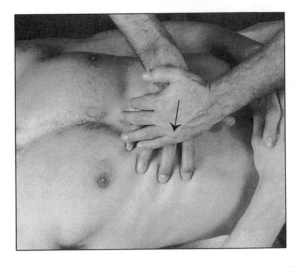
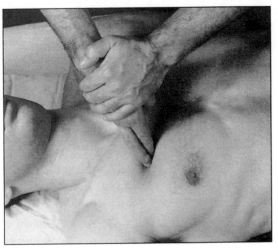

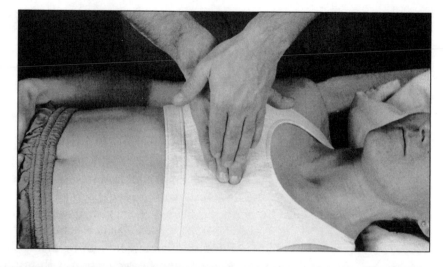

Deep friction can be applied through clothing into the sternocostal space, which can have an effect along the intercostal muscle running under the breast tissue.

Accessory breathing muscles

	MUSCLE	ACTION
Exhalation	Abdominal muscles	Increases abdominal pressure
	Serratus anterior	Draws shoulders forward
	Pectoralis major	
	Quadratus lumborum	Lowers ribcage as diaphragm raises
Inhalation	Scalenes	Raises upper ribs
	Trapezius	Draws back scapula
	Rhomboids	
	Levator scapula	Elevates scapula
	Serratus posterior	Draws back ribs
	Sternocleidomastoid	Raises upper ribs
	Pectoralis minor	

An efficient breathing pattern needs freedom of movement in the ribcage and shoulders, and any muscle tension or structural imbalance that restricts this can be detrimental. All the muscles of the torso can therefore be considered as having some involvement in the breathing process.

These accessory muscles are dealt with elsewhere, according to their primary function.

Shoulders

Shoulder movements are made through two articulating structures: the shoulder girdle and the shoulder joint itself. The girdle articulates on two joints; one lies between the sternum and clavicle (sternoclavicular) and the other between the acromion process of the scapula and the clavicle (acromioclavicular). The third and most mobile structure is the ball-and-socket joint between the glenoid cavity of the scapula and the humerus (glenohumeral). The scapula does not directly articulate with any other bones and has considerable mobility, due to the action of many muscles. All the upper back muscles, therefore, are involved to some extent in moving the shoulder girdle.

Normal function requires all these structures to work in an integrated way, and any restriction in either the joint or the girdle will lead to some over-use in the other. The original restriction may develop very slowly and go unnoticed, and discomfort could first be felt in the secondary area suffering the over-use.

Many of the shoulder muscles have close or common attachments around the upper part of the humerus, and injury or tension in one muscle often produces referred symptoms in another. This is why patients often have difficulty in locating the actual point of pain. For this reason, all the shoulder muscles should be assessed carefully whenever treating a shoulder problem, even when the painful symptoms can easily be identified.

With so many muscles involved in all movements, a minor injury to only a small muscle can cause considerable dysfunction. Other muscles rapidly weaken through lack of use, so strength exercises are always an important part of rehabilitation.

Trapezius

MUSCLE	ORIGIN	INSERTION	ACTION
Trapezius	Occipital bone, ligaments of cervical spine and thoracic spine	Clavicle and spine of scapula	Stabilizes scapula, and some elevation and rotation

This is the large muscle that overlies many other muscles in the upper back and neck area and has several functions. It is often considered in two halves: the upper part, which attaches to the base of the skull and moves the head and neck; and the lower part, which draws the scapula together and downwards. The key function of the muscle as a whole is to control and stabilize the scapula in all neck and shoulder movements.

The trapezius does not commonly suffer acute strain as smaller, more specific muscles normally get damaged first, but a build-up of tension and fibrosis are quite common. This is often associated with

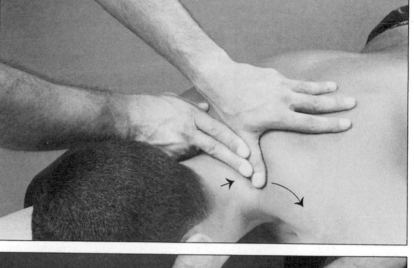

Deep stroking with the
thumb along the upper
trapezius muscle.

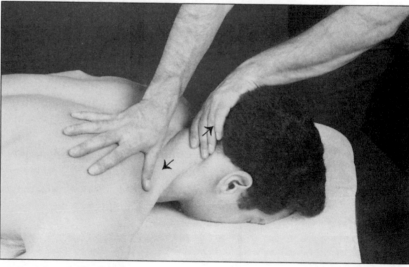

Stroking and stretching
the upper trapezius at the
same time.

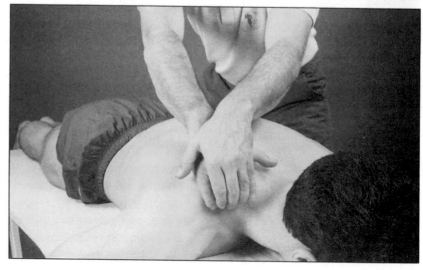

With the fingers hooked
around the muscle, the
tips of the fingers can
press into the anterior
trapezius fibres and apply
stroking and friction
techniques.

problems in deeper muscles and is usually due to repetitive over-use and postural factors. The upper fibres running laterally out to the acromion process (top of the shoulders) are most often affected in this way because of a raised or hunched shoulder position. The muscle usually feels hard and dense here, or in other parts of the trapezius, where the fibres have matted together through constant shortening of the fibres (postural) and/or scar tissue and adhesions from micro-trauma (over-use).

Increased curvature (lordosis) in the cervical spine can make the trapezius actually look like two muscles, as a distinct crease can develop across the fibres at the base of the neck. This will affect the function of the whole muscle, especially the upper part, and restricts blood circulation, which can contribute to headaches. The crease also suggests that the cervical curvature is fairly extreme and putting con-siderable stress on the lower cervical vertebrae. Even though the patient may not be aware of a spinal problem, palpation around these bones may be quite painful. The tissues surrounding them will feel thick and congested, and gentle friction can help release this. Loosening the fibrous tissue and stretching out this crease is vital if any postural improvement is to be achieved.

Treatment
Specific treatment of the trapezius can be carried out in the prone posi-tion, with a cushion under the patient's shoulders to flex the neck and open out the area. Treatment methods for the upper part of the muscle are the same as for the other posterior neck muscles, but particular attention should be paid to the lateral fibres running out to the shoul-der joint. Deep squeezing and petrissage, as well as deep friction with NMT (see Chapter 14) and stretching, all work very well here.

The lower part of the muscle between the scapula lies over the rhomboid muscles and the two are generally treated together (see p.133).

Levator scapula			
MUSCLE	ORIGIN	INSERTION	ACTION
Levator scapula	C1 to C4	Superior angle of scapula	Raises scapula or rotates and side-bends head

As well as elevating the scapula when the shoulders are fixed, the leva-tor scapula acts to move the head (the role of the origin and insertion being reversed). Its most usual function, however, is in stabilizing the neck and shoulders by preventing the scapula from being pulled down when the arms are weighted. It is therefore put under stress in many lifting activities, particularly in people with hunched shoulders. This control function often requires a static or slightly eccentric contraction, which is more likely to cause micro-trauma. Scar tissue is commonly found to build up around the scapula attachment.

Treatment

This muscle is generally treated along with the posterior neck muscles in prone or supine positions. Strokes should also be made down the neck to the scapula attachment, where deep friction can help break down the scar tissue. Stretching is also extremely important.

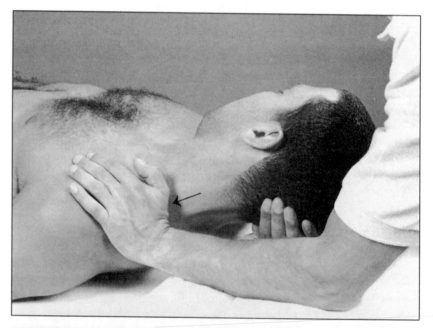

In the supine position, the head can be supported in a slight flexion and rotation, while the other hand can apply a stroke along the levator scapula.

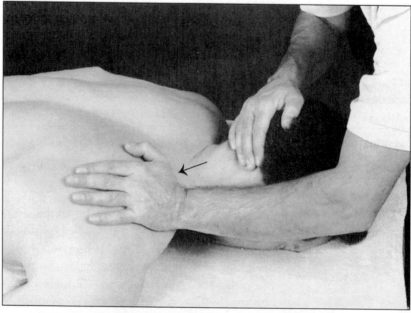

In the prone position, one hand fixes the position of the head to prevent the muscle from shortening, and a stroke can be applied down to the scapula attachment.

Rhomboid muscles

MUSCLE	ORIGIN	INSERTION	ACTION
Rhomboid minor	C6 and C7	Medial border of scapula	Braces scapula and draws it medially and downwards
Rhomboid major	T1 to T4		

These are deep muscles that run from the vertebrae, diagonally downwards to the scapula. They are important postural muscles, which help maintain the position of the scapula. They are commonly found to be posturally weak and stretched, due to the opposing action of short, tight pectoral muscles in the front of the chest. This can be visibly noticeable, with the shoulder-blades protruding from the surface of the back along their medial borders.

The action of pulling the shoulder-blades together is not a common voluntary action and is seldom done with any great force, so acute strain is rare. The rhomboid muscles are more involved in controlling or preventing the scapula from moving down and outwards when holding a heavy object. They are therefore more likely to suffer from a build-up of tension through gradual over-use, especially if the muscle is also posturally weak. Micro-trauma tends to occur more along the attachment with the scapula, and fibrous adhesions often build up here. Injury to this muscle may cause painful symptoms to be referred into the chest area.

Treatment

Deep stroking with the forearm to the lower trapezius and rhomboid muscles.

Once the overlying trapezius muscle has been softened, stroking techniques to the rhomboids should be applied diagonally across the body in opposite directions, to treat the fibres longitudinally and transversely. Friction can be applied to any local area of tension in the muscles in the normal prone position, but to treat the scapula border the 'scapula lift' (see p.136) position can be used. Deep friction around the vertebral attachments can release tension throughout the thoracic area, as well as in the muscle itself.

The pectoral muscles must be assessed along with the rhomboids to restore good balance between them.

The *serratus posterior superior* lies beneath the rhomboids and attaches to the ribs under the scapula. It raises the ribs and is a respiratory muscle assisting inhalation. It is treated together with the rhomboids.

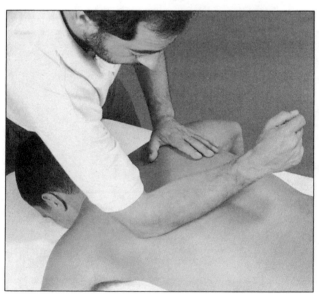

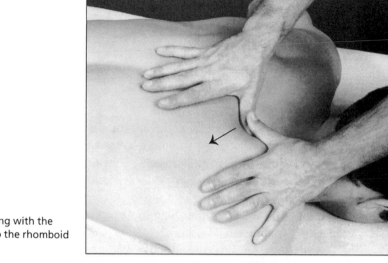

Deep stroking with the thumbs into the rhomboid muscle.

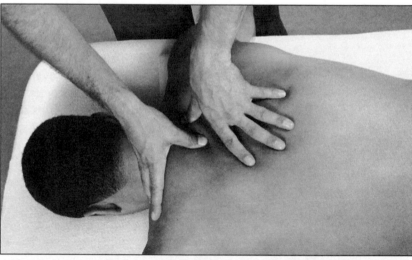

Friction with the thumbs into the muscle origins of the lower trapezius and rhomboid muscles and ligaments around the vertebrae.

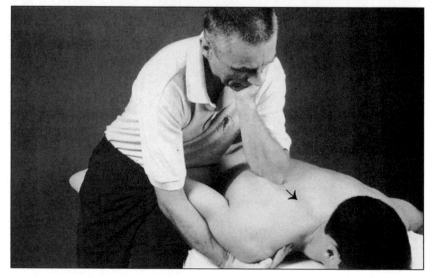

Deep friction and stroking into the rhomboid muscle using the elbow. The shoulder is lifted to raise the medial border of the scapula, and the stroke can then be guided along this edge.

Serratus anterior			
MUSCLE	ORIGIN	INSERTION	ACTION
Serratus anterior	Lateral surface of 1st to 12th ribs	Anterior surface of medial border of scapula	Draws scapula forward (protracts) and rotates it

The main function of this muscle is to move the scapula forward and up, which is one of the principal components in raising the arm. As this moves the scapula in the opposite direction to the rhomboids, these two muscles work together to control its position.

It is not often injured, but since it is attached to the ribs, tension can build up in association with other chest muscles. In activities such as swimming or climbing, this muscle can become damaged through overuse, and it is important to treat it as part of any general massage for people involved in these types of activities.

Treatment

As most of the muscle lies between the shoulder-blade and ribs, it is difficult to reach without specially positioning the patient. Side-lying the patient with his upper arm abducted over the side of the head, the therapist can apply stroking techniques to the lateral fibres, below the armpit. In the supine position the arm can be fully abducted to draw the scapula out from the ribs. The therapist's fingers can then stroke and friction between the ribs and the scapula, and towards the muscle insertion.

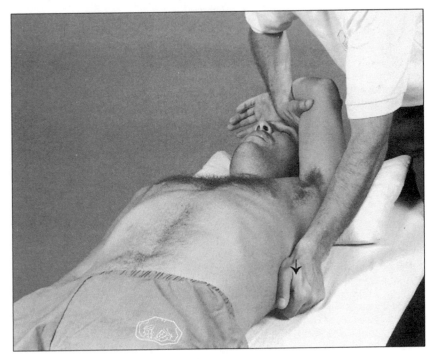

With the arm held in abduction, stroking can be applied into the serratus anterior muscle with the heel of the hand.

With the patient in a side-lying position with the arm abducted, the heel of the therapist's hand and thumb can stroke through the serratus anterior muscle.

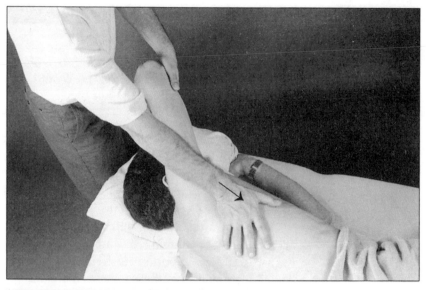

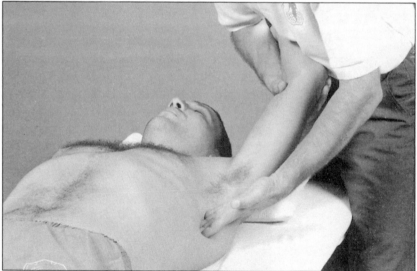

The fingertips can work around the ribs to friction the serratus anterior fibres beneath the scapula.

Scapula lift

The scapula does not articulate with any bones of the trunk, and its position is maintained by the many muscles that attach to it. It needs to be able to move freely to enable all the muscles to function in an integrated way, and a problem in one muscle can affect the function of the rest. The therapist needs to be able to lift and move the scapula around to get better access to the surrounding tissues and particularly the muscles that lie underneath it (serratus anterior and subscapularis).

To do this, the patient should be in a prone position with the arm resting across his lower back (or by his side if more comfortable). The therapist can then put one hand round the front of the shoulder joint and pull it upwards. Unless the upper back and chest muscles are very tight, this should raise the whole scapula away from the underlying ribs.

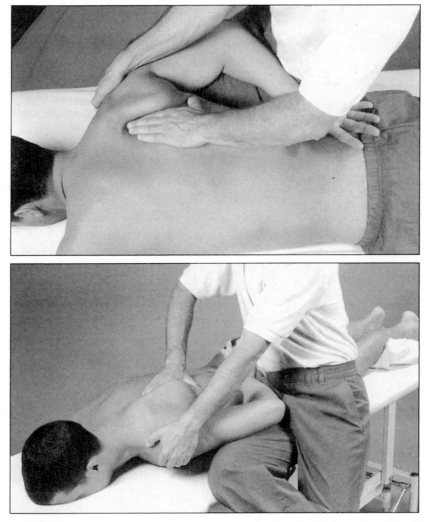

Right (above and below): Grasping around the front of the shoulder, the therapist can lean back to lift the scapula. The other hand can then be used to stroke and friction the tissues underneath the bone.

Below: In the scapula lift position, with one hand grasping the shoulder joint and the other fixed around the superior angle of the scapula. The bone can be glided in all lateral directions to stretch many of the upper back muscles.

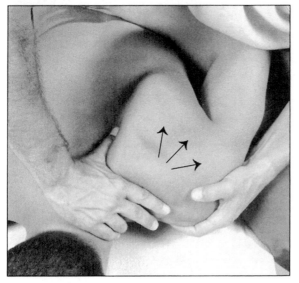

The fingers and thumb of the other hand can then work the tissues under and around the borders of the bone. The fingers can press passively into the tissues, with frictional movement being made with the other hand pulling the scapula over the fingers. Alternatively, the scapula can be held still while the fingers apply the friction; or the two can be combined.

If the tissues relax sufficiently, the fingers can ease their way in very deeply behind the scapula. Here friction can be applied downwards to the ribs, intercostal muscles and serratus anterior, or up against the surface of the scapula to treat the subscapularis.

To stretch

With one hand lifting the shoulder joint, the other hand can fit around the medial and superior borders of the scapula. In this position the therapist has a firm grip, with the whole of the scapula between his hands, and it can then be moved in all directions to stretch the surrounding tissues (see lower example on p.137).

If the muscles are extremely tense, the most powerful way of applying a scapula lift is with the patient in the side-lying position, facing the therapist and with his arm resting behind his back. The therapist puts one hand through the gap between the arm and chest, and curls the fingers up behind the medial border of the scapula. The fingers of the other hand can be inserted next to them. The therapist can then use his body to push down on the shoulder and move the scapula over the fingers as they apply a deep friction.

To stretch the muscles, particularly the rhomboids, the whole shoulder girdle can be locked between the therapist's hands and body and lifted up, away from the spine. To do this the couch needs to be very low so that the therapist can bend his knees and use his hip against the front of the patient's shoulder. By standing up it is actually possible to lift a patient off the couch by their scapula. (This should only be done if the muscles are very tight. If they are relaxed, the force of this technique could cause them to tear.)

With the patient in a side-lying position, the therapist can grasp around the medial border of the scapula and lift it away from the body to stretch excessively tight rhomboid muscles.

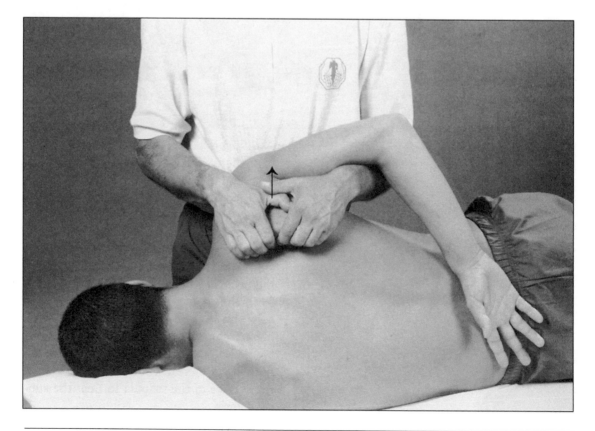

Adductors of the arm

MUSCLE	ORIGIN	INSERTION	ACTION
Latissimus dorsi	T7 to T12, and via lumbar fascia to L1 to L5 and iliac crest	Bicipital groove of humerus	Adducts, draws back (extends) and inwardly rotates arm
Teres major	Lower lateral border of scapula	Medial lip of bicipital groove of humerus	Inwardly rotates and adducts arm

The *latissimus dorsi* is a superficial muscle that covers most of the lower half of the back but is actually a shoulder muscle. It is the most powerful adductor muscle of the arm, and also inwardly rotates and pulls the arm back. It is, therefore, a major muscle in many powerful arm and shoulder activities, such as swimming or climbing.

It is naturally a strong, flexible muscle, and acute injury tends to occur only with very extreme effort. Areas of tension and fibrosis can sometimes be felt along the outer border, which tends to take more of the force, due to micro-trauma in over-use situations. Although the latissimus dorsi is a large muscle with considerable strength, the force of contraction is focused on a small area of attachment at the humerus. Micro-trauma is more likely to occur here as the fibres are put under greater stress.

Treatment

To treat the latissimus dorsi in the prone position, the patient's arm should be abducted to enable deep longitudinal strokes all the way from the lower back to the insertion at the armpit (axilla). Deep transverse strokes can be applied with the therapist standing on the opposite site of the couch, curling his fingers round the lateral border of the muscle and then pulling back across the fibres. Friction around the insertion can be carried out along with the teres insertion, when the arm is abducted.

The *posterior inferior serratus* muscle lies beneath the latissimus dorsi and attaches to the lower ribs. Drawing them downwards, it is a respiratory muscle assisting in inspiration. It is treated together with the latissimus dorsi origin area.

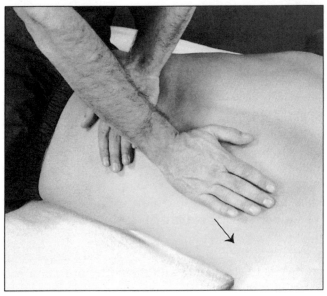

Long stroking with the palm working up the latissimus dorsi muscle.

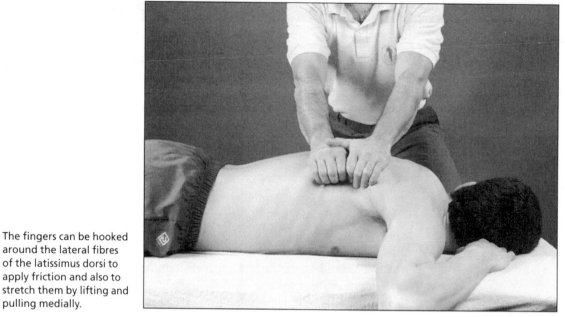

The fingers can be hooked around the lateral fibres of the latissimus dorsi to apply friction and also to stretch them by lifting and pulling medially.

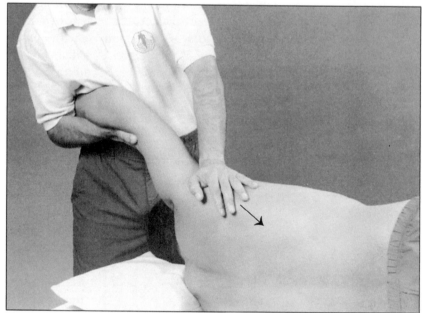

With the patient side-lying with the arm abducted, one hand can apply a stroke through the adductor muscles, and the other hand can increase the stretch by further abducting the patient's arm.

The *teres major* muscle is a smaller muscle, which lies beneath the latissimus dorsi and runs from the lower lateral border of the scapula diagonally upwards. It passes in front of the long head of the triceps muscle and attaches anteriorly round the humerus, so it is an inward rotator as well as a strong adductor of the arm.

Treatment

The teres major muscle is treated along with the posterior rotator cuff muscles and the latissimus dorsi.

Rotator cuff muscles

MUSCLE	ORIGIN	INSERTION	ACTION
Supraspinatus	Upper dorsal surface of scapula	Great tuberosity of humerus	Abducts arm
Infraspinatus	Lower dorsal surface of scapula		Outwardly rotates arm
Teres minor	Lateral border of scapula		
Subscapularis	Anterior surface of scapula	Lesser tuberosity of humerus	Inwardly rotates arm

To allow the great range of movement capable in the glenohumeral joint, its socket is very shallow, which also makes it relatively unstable. The rotator cuff muscles that attach around the upper part of the humerus hold the ball and socket in place and keep the joint stable. A structural joint problem will affect these muscles but, more commonly, an injury to one of the muscles will affect the joint's stability, which can lead to other problems.

The joint is commonly sprained, or even dislocated, when it is forced through an extreme range. As well as tearing the ligaments, the rotator cuff muscles will nearly always be damaged too. When putting the arm out to protect a fall, the impact is forced up through the humerus and pushes it out from the socket, and can also strain or over-stretch the muscles. Following such injuries it is vital to strengthen these muscles to restore joint stability and prevent a recurrence.

Over-use injuries can be quite common in throwing activities, and inflammation can occur at the insertions. Even though the muscles are at the back, painful symptoms may appear to come from the front of the shoulder or even down the arm. Injury to the rotator cuff muscles is often mistaken for 'frozen shoulder' (see p.150).

The *supraspinatus* has a special function, as it provides the first few degrees of abduction in the arm, at which point the deltoid muscle takes over the action. It is the only muscle of the group to have its origin above the spine of the scapula, and only this part of it can be palpated, as the rest of the muscle runs behind the acromion. Repetitive shoulder actions with the arm raised high can cause the tendon of this muscle to get pinched above the humeral head, which can cause it to become inflamed (tendonitis).

The *infraspinatus* muscle runs along the inferior border of the spine of the scapula and runs *posterially* to the great tuberosity.

The origin of the teres minor muscle is at the lateral border of the scapula and it lies partly beneath the infraspinatus. It runs diagonally upwards and attaches *posterially* to the humerus and so *outwardly* rotates it, as well as assisting slightly in adduction.

The *subscapularis* is completely hidden beneath the scapula and can only be reached in the 'scapula lift' position (see p.136). It inserts at the lesser tuberosity, which is *anterior* and so creates *inward* rotation. It is also important in controlling and preventing excessive outward rotation and can become chronically tense if over-used in this situation. This muscle is also often the first to become affected as a secondary symptom in the 'frozen shoulder' condition. Tension in this muscle can sometimes lead to referred symptoms in the front of the chest.

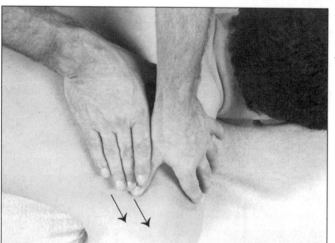

Deep stroking and friction with the thumb towards the insertions of the posterior rotator cuff muscles.

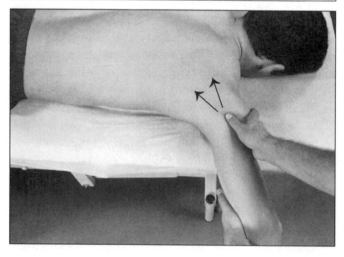

With the arm held in an abducted position, deep strokes can be applied with the thumb from the insertion towards the origins of the rotator cuff muscles.

Treatment

To treat the rotator cuff muscles, long strokes can be applied from the medial scapula border out to the insertions at the back of the shoulder. Deeper strokes can be better applied in the other direction, with the therapist standing to the side of the couch. The patient's arm can be held in abduction with one hand, while the other can apply deep friction into areas of damage within the group.

The posterior insertions at the head of the humerus can be palpated by working the fingers or thumbs under the posterior border of the deltoid muscle. Deep friction may require both thumbs, and in order to maintain relaxed abduction of the patient's arm the therapist can use the outside of his thigh to prevent it moving.

The muscles can be treated in a side-lying position along with the serratus anterior. The anterior attachments around the humerus should be treated with friction when the patient is in the supine position. The arm should be comfortably supported by the therapist and moved into different positions to assess and treat the area thoroughly.

In the supine position, the patient's arm can be fully abducted so that the scapula is drawn out from behind the ribs. From here, friction can be applied down onto the anterior surface of the bone and in towards its attachment (similar to the serratus anterior position).

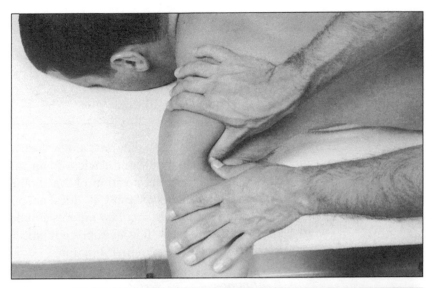

Friction with the thumbs into the posterior insertions of the rotator cuff muscles.

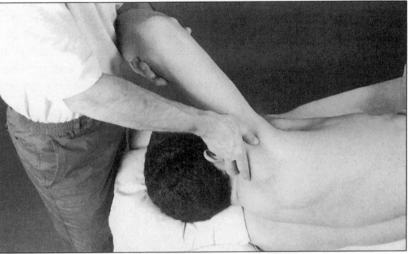

In a side-lying position with the arm abducted, deep friction can be applied into the rotator cuff insertions and around the joint capsule.

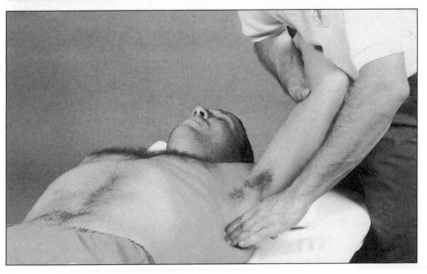

In the supine position with the arm abducted, the therapist's fingers can friction down onto the subscapularis muscle.

Subclavicular muscle

MUSCLE	ORIGIN	INSERTION	ACTION
Subclavicular	Medial end of 1st rib	Inferior surface of clavicle	Draws shoulder girdle forward and down

This is a thin muscle, which runs along the clavicle bone and is mostly hidden beneath it. It pulls the clavicle down and so stabilizes the sterno-clavicular joint and the position of the shoulder girdle. Although discomfort is rarely felt locally, it does become chronically tense in association with other shoulder injuries and postural imbalances in the upper torso and neck. It is an important muscle to treat as it can significantly affect overall shoulder function.

Treatment

To treat the muscle, deep strokes can be made along the posterior border of the bone and should go deeper under the bone as it moves out towards the shoulder joint. Friction can be applied transversely to the fibres by applying short, deep strokes up behind the bone. Sometimes it is necessary to work from above the bone and apply friction down behind it.

The subclavicular muscle can be reached with friction and stroking under the clavicle bone.

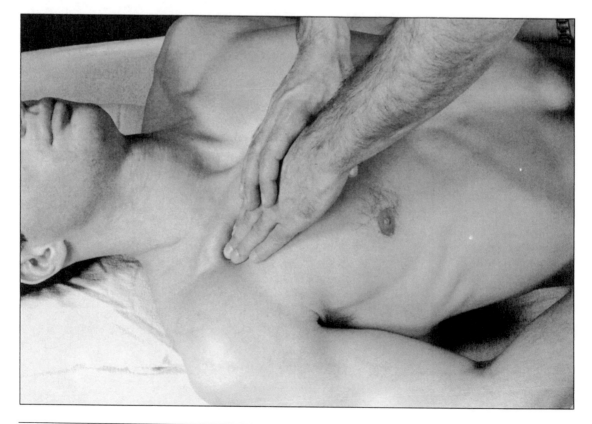

Pectorals			
MUSCLE	ORIGIN	INSERTION	ACTION
Pectoralis major	Clavicle, sternum, 1st to 6th ribs, abdominal aponeurosis and obliques	Lateral lip of bicipital groove of humerus	Horizontal adduction, adducts, flexes and inwardly rotates arm
Pectoralis minor	3rd to 5th ribs	Coracoid process of scapula	Draws scapula forward and down

The *pectoralis major* is a very large muscle divided into many compartments. As these compartments converge towards the insertion, they twist round so that the lower fibres insert above the fibres that come down from the clavicle. This not only maintains the shape of the muscle, but also gives it considerable strength through a wide range of abduction and rotational movements.

Injury, or increased tension through over-use, tends to occur in individual compartments, depending on the particular range of movement involved.

Protracted (forwardly rotated) shoulders, which form a very common postural imbalance, can cause the muscle as a whole to shorten (see also rhomboids on p.133).

Imbalance is often found within the muscle due to poor training. Strength exercises for the pectorals are often done through only one or two ranges, which will leave some parts of the muscle unaffected. Without correct supervision, some people with protracted shoulders will exercise the pectorals very hard, but improving their flexibility instead would be more beneficial. And if they do not counteract this by also strengthening the rhomboid muscles, then they can make the postural imbalance worse.

The *pectoralis minor* muscle lies beneath the pectoralis major and is much smaller and has a significantly different function. Although it is considered a shoulder joint muscle, it does not attach to the humerus like the others.

In normal activities, with the arm down, the muscle has no real involvement. But when the arm is raised above the head it is lengthened and its main purpose is then to pull the shoulder back to a normal position as part of the overall downward arm action. It can therefore become injured through over-use or over-stretching in activities like tennis that involve a lot of overhead arm action. The muscle also becomes shorter with a protracted shoulder position, which can add to the risk of injury.

It is hard to identify this muscle as the source of pain, as symptoms tend to spread into the larger pectoralis major muscle or into the shoulder.

Treatment

Tension and micro-trauma can develop anywhere in the pectoralis major muscle due to over-use, and the muscle must be assessed thoroughly to find areas that may require deeper friction. The arm needs to be abducted to allow long strokes from the sternum to reach the insertion, which is under the anterior border of the deltoid. Deep stroking and friction can be used on local areas of tension and fibrosis.

It is only possible to identify the pectoralis minor muscle when the overlying muscle has been softened and relaxed. Slightly stretching it, by raising the arm over the head, will make it stand out more clearly. In this position friction can be applied to the origins through the softer superficial muscle, and long strokes can follow the fibres up to the top of the shoulder. Friction can be applied wherever necessary.

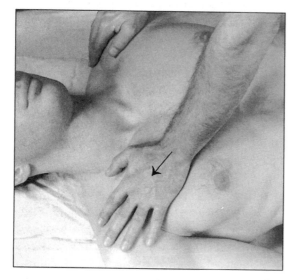 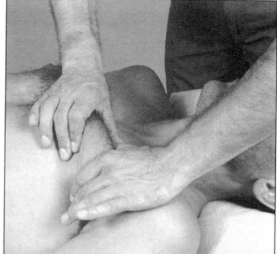

Above: Stroking with the heel of the palm towards the insertion of the pectoralis major.

Above (right): Kneading (petrissage) to the pectoralis major.

Right: With the arm extended above the head, the fingers can friction the pectoralis minor through the major muscle.

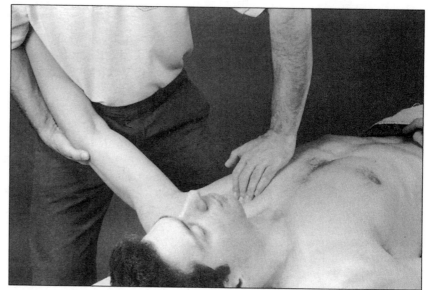

Deltoid

MUSCLE	ORIGIN	INSERTION	ACTION
Deltoid	Clavicle, acromion and spine of scapula	Deltoid tuberosity of humerus (midway along)	Anterior: draws arm forward and inwardly rotates Lateral: abducts arm Posterior: draws arm back (extends) and outwardly rotates

This is the large, rounded muscle that wraps around the outside of the shoulder. It is made up of many compartments, which together enable the muscle to raise the arm to about 90 degrees forward, sideways and backwards.

Individual compartments can become tense through repetitive use or over-use, depending on the particular range of movement involved. Some imbalance is natural as compartments will develop according to use, and the anterior part is usually the strongest since most actions tend to be made with the arms out in front of the body.

All the compartments converge into a small area of attachment halfway down the lateral shaft of the humerus. Tension often builds up here, and the tissues can thicken with fibrous adhesions.

Treatment

The posterior part of the muscle can be treated in the prone position, but the whole muscle can be worked easily from the supine position. The therapist should sit on the edge of the couch facing the patient's

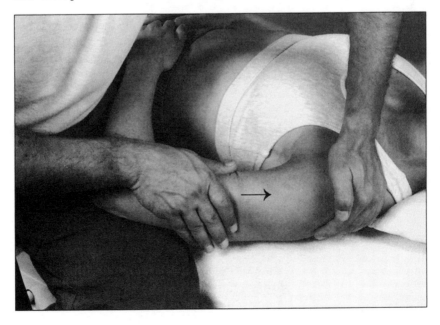

With one hand on top of the shoulder joint to prevent movement, the other hand can apply strokes up through the deltoid muscle.

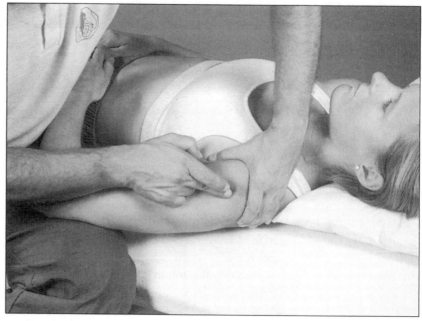

The fingertips can be used to friction into the deltoid muscle.

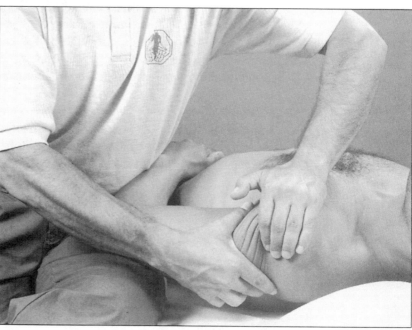

Kneading (petrissage) of the deltoid muscle.

head, with the patient's elbow resting on the therapist's thigh, which lifts the shoulder. In this position the hands can reach all round the muscle and treat each compartment. Friction should be applied wherever tight or congested areas are felt.

The subdeltoid bursa is located just below the great tubercle of the humerus, beneath the lateral deltoid. It can become inflamed (bursitis) through impact injury, but symptoms will appear to suggest a muscle injury.

Coracobrachialis

MUSCLE	ORIGIN	INSERTION	ACTION
Coracobrachialis	Coracoid process of scapula	Medial border of humerus (midway along)	Draws arm forward and inward

This is a small muscle running from deep within the front of the shoulder, down the inside of the biceps tendon, and it attaches midway down the humerus. The forward and medially rotated arm position created by this muscle is one that is commonly used in everyday activities, and over-used in racket sports. Whenever the arms are being held out in front of the body, the coracobrachialis is one of the main muscles involved. As these positions are often held statically for long periods, for instance when driving, the constant isometric contraction often leads to this muscle becoming tense and fibrous. Painful symptoms are usually felt in the shoulder.

Treatment

The coracobrachialis can be treated in the same position as that used for the deltoid. As it is normally found to be hard and congested, it is usually quite easy to identify and treat with deep stroking and friction. Initial treatment can have a considerable effect but may cause residual pain for a few days. Stretching exercises, with the arm back behind the body, are important if treatment is to be successful.

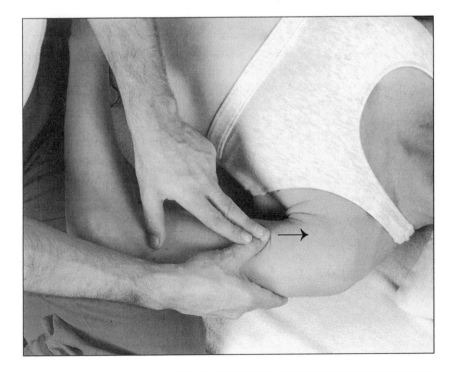

Deep stroking up the coracobrachialis muscle with the thumb.

'Frozen shoulder' (adhesive capsulitis)

This is a condition that causes considerable pain and great dysfunction, and tends to occur in people over 40 and is more common in women.

The synovial capsule surrounding the glenohumeral joint is a very loose one, especially on the inferior side, where it has to accommodate up to 180 degrees of abduction. When the arm is down, the capsule folds in, and if the capsule is not regularly stretched, creases can form in the synovial membrane, which may become adhered and inflamed. In everyday life we regularly move the arm above the shoulder when taking things off a shelf or even when sleeping. But if this does not happen naturally, or when movement is restricted for a period of time by another injury, the 'frozen shoulder' condition can arise.

Symptoms usually appear suddenly one morning, and because even a small adhesion will affect the function of the whole synovial membrane, pain and dysfunction can be severe. Through lack of use over time, the rotator cuff muscles, particularly the subscapularis, rapidly weaken and become tense. This adds to the poor function, which prevents any functional stretching that might help release the adhesions and stop any more developing. Over time the whole capsule, and the fluid within it, can thicken.

Symptoms may persist for several months, and when the adhesion does eventually release, recovery can be just as sudden as the condition's onset. Sometimes, however, this is not actually noticed at the time, because the muscle dysfunction has become so great that it causes the same symptoms.

Treatment

Massage treatment can have little direct effect on the capsulitis itself as it is only possible to reach the affected tissue in a few isolated spots. It can deal only with the secondary muscular component of the condition.

By treating all the associated muscles and generally stimulating the circulation through the joint, the symptoms should at least stabilize and at best this treatment may help facilitate recovery.

Active and passive exercises, through as full a range of movement as possible, are an important part of treatment of this condition. They will help prevent muscle dysfunction and may help release the capsular adhesion.

When treating a shoulder injury in people over 40, especially women, the possibility of it developing into a 'frozen shoulder' should be considered. Patients should be encouraged to continue regular treatment and to perform overarm exercises until their injury has been completely resolved.

Other shoulder injuries, including a simple muscle strain, are often mis-diagnosed as being a 'frozen shoulder' since they may have similar symptoms.

The arm

Biceps brachii			
MUSCLE	ORIGIN	INSERTION	ACTION
Biceps brachii	Long head: passes over top of joint to supraglenoid tubercle of scapula Short head: coracoid process of scapula	Via a strong tendon to radial tuberosity and bicipital aponeurosis	Strong: flexor and supinator of forearm Weak: abducts and inwardly rotates arm (long head) Adducts arm (short head)

This is the large muscle of the upper arm most noted as the powerful flexor of the elbow, but it is actually a two-joint muscle, which also assists shoulder movement and forearm supination. When lifting a heavy object, the elbow and shoulder move together, as the biceps muscle is primarily involved. It also assists in supination of the lower arm, which is functionally a more powerful action than pronation.

The biceps brachii is a purely voluntary muscle, which gets heavily used in many activities. Although it responds well to strength training, it commonly becomes strained with repetitive use or overload. It has a rich blood supply and is easy to rest when injured, so it usually recovers quickly. However, holding the muscle in a shortened position to aid recovery can lead to the tissues remaining short and tight afterwards.

Chronic shortening of the muscle is sometimes seen in people who subject it to heavy loading without proper stretching. A muscle produces its greatest force in its inner range, and in an effort to lift greater weight the individual has to limit movement to within that range. Without proper stretching of the muscle afterwards, it can permanently shorten, eventually, and full elbow extension then becomes impossible.

The tendon at the insertion into the lower arm is very strong, and a considerable force of contraction converges into it from the muscle. Scar tissue from micro-trauma is therefore most likely to develop here, around the muscle tendon junction.

The muscle has two tendon heads, the longer one passing over the top of the head of the humerus and through the joint, to attach above the glenoid cavity (joint socket). Repetitive muscle contraction in conjunction with a high arm and shoulder movements can cause this tendon to rub against the bony joint structures and become inflamed (tendonitis). This is a common cause of shoulder pain, and the whole muscle needs to be treated as well as the local area of pain. Occasionally the tendon of the long head can slip round to the front of the joint, if its retaining ligament becomes stretched. Although this may not cause much pain, it needs to be medically assessed as massage can do nothing to relocate it.

Treatment

The belly of the biceps muscle can be treated with the patient's elbow slightly flexed, to shorten and relax it, but the elbow must be extended to allow friction around the distal insertion. Stroking up the muscle, the therapist's fingers or thumbs can follow the fibres up into the tendons and trace their path under the deltoid (which needs to be softened first) through to their insertion. Any points along the tendons that feel thick, tense or painful should be treated gently with friction techniques. It is advisable to ice the tendon after treatment, especially in post-acute conditions. To reach the deeper muscle fibres, friction can be applied transversely from the side to work between the muscle and the bone.

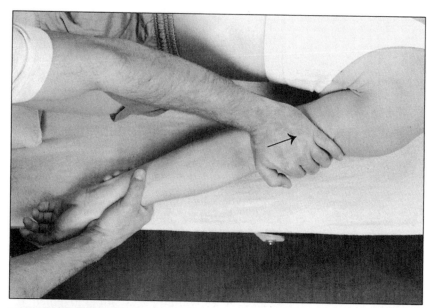

Stroking along the biceps brachii muscle with the heel of the palm.

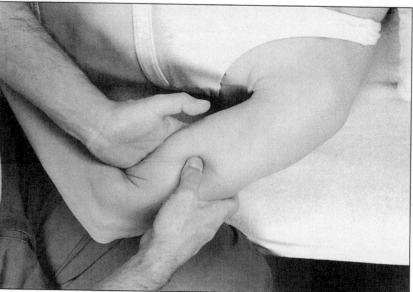

With one hand lifting the biceps muscle, friction can be applied with the thumb into the deep fibres close to the bone.

Brachialis			
MUSCLE	ORIGIN	INSERTION	ACTION
Brachialis	Lower anterior surface of humerus	Ulnar tuberosity	Flexes forearm

This is the main flexor of the elbow joint when lifting a small load. It runs down between the lateral border of the biceps and the humerus to the elbow. Only when the brachialis reaches its maximum force does the biceps become involved, and shoulder movement and supination of the lower arm usually occur also.

The origin of the muscle attaches to a very large area over the humerus, but it has only a small insertion into the ulna, so over-use tension is more likely here, with pain resulting in the elbow. The brachialis is commonly found to be slightly tight in people who use a lot of powerful elbow flexion in their sport or occupation (such as massage therapy). This can be visibly observed in the elbow, which remains slightly flexed when the arm is resting down by the side; but it can be fully extended by contracting the triceps (if it is the biceps that are short, the elbow will not extend fully).

Treatment

To treat this muscle the patient's elbow should be slightly flexed and the arm inwardly rotated. Deep stroking techniques can be applied with the thumb or fingers from the elbow up through the muscle. Any areas of tension can be treated with friction, which can be applied from the lateral side under the biceps. To reach the insertion, the elbow should be more flexed and the fingers can then palpate and friction the surface of the ulna on the inside of the joint.

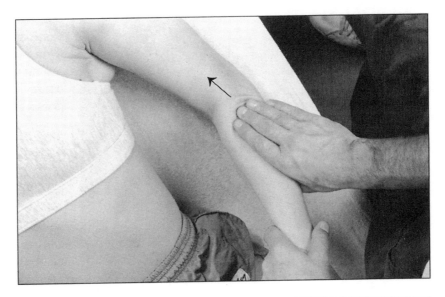

With the elbow slightly flexed by elevating the forearm, the other hand can be used to stroke and friction the brachialis muscle.

Triceps brachii

MUSCLE	ORIGIN	INSERTION	ACTION
Triceps brachii	Long head: infra-glenoid tubercle of scapula Medial and lateral heads: posterior surface of humerus	Through a flat tendon to the olecranon process of ulna	Extends elbow Long head: adducts arm

The medial and lateral heads of this muscle have their origins covering a large area of the dorsal surface of the humerus, but the long head originates from a small area on the scapula. The long head is therefore a two-joint muscle, which assists shoulder adduction as well as combining with the other two parts to extend the elbow.

In normal activities the triceps are often working in a gravity-assisted situation and do not require great strength. But there are many sports, like swimming and boxing, and occupational activities, like massage, that require strong elbow extension. The muscle does strengthen very well in response to use but can be injured through over-use. It can become weak in response to an over-development of strength in the biceps, which will increase its vulnerability to injury.

Due to the range of flexion possible at the elbow joint, it is not feasible to stretch the muscle fully through normal use. So with repetitive over-use, tension can develop that does not naturally get a chance to be stretched and released. This tension is usually felt along the muscle tendon junctions towards the elbow.

With the arm extended above the head, the triceps can be treated with the thumb.

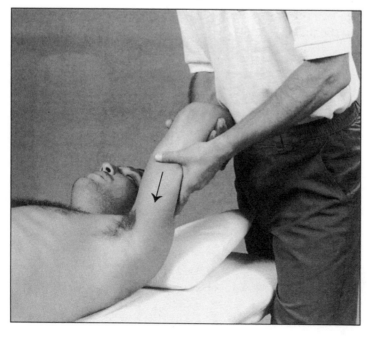

The large, flat tendon through which the triceps brachii inserts frequently gets damaged through impact. Scar tissue and fibrous adhesions that form in the tendon can affect the function of the muscles and cause pain generally in the dorsal part of the elbow.

Treatment
The muscle can be treated in the prone position with the patient's forearm hanging down off the side of the couch. Long strokes, with friction where necessary, can be applied from the elbow up towards the origins beneath the posterior deltoid.

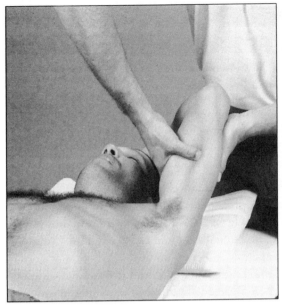

Friction can be applied with the thumb into the deep fibres close to the bone.

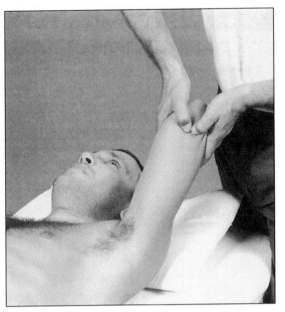

Deep friction with the thumbs to the triceps tendon.

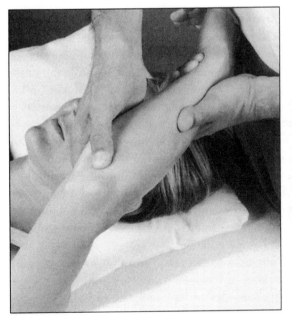

Friction around the elbow joint in the supine and prone positions.

Deeper treatment can be given in the supine position with the patient's arm extended over his head and supported by the therapist (standing at the head) holding it just above the elbows, so that the patient's forearm hangs down. The therapist's other hand can be used to apply deep strokes along the muscle. Friction can be applied in from the sides to reach the deepest fibres and attachments along the bone.

Forearm (radial side)

MUSCLE	ORIGIN	INSERTION	ACTION
Brachioradialis	Distal, lateral edge of humerus	Distal, lateral surface of radius	Flexes forearm
Common extensors	Lateral epicondyle of humerus	Base of metacarpals and phalanges	Extends and abducts/adducts wrist and hand

With the elbow slightly flexed, radial side up, the brachioradialis is the large muscle uppermost. The forearm is neither pronated nor supinated in this position, and this muscle becomes the main elbow flexor. The common extensor muscles lie beneath it and run through long tendons into the thumb and forefinger.

Many sport, occupational and leisure activities involve the action of these muscles, which get heavily used. They often become tense due to over-use, which can lead to the extremely common 'tennis elbow' condition.

'Tennis elbow' (lateral epicondylitis)

The radial forearm muscles respond well to use and become quite strong, but the force of contraction is focused on a very small area of attachment at the humerus. The tissues here are put under great stress to cope with the load, so micro-trauma can occur and lead to a build-up of fibrous tissue. This reduces the elasticity of the tissues, which increases the pull on the attachments and can make the problem worse.

These muscles are often involved in activities that require them to perform a braking action to prevent movement in the elbow and wrist. When hitting a tennis ball or digging, for example, the elbow and wrist joints remain virtually fixed and the muscles have to resist a sudden force. This type of sharp, eccentric contraction can be highly damaging to the tissues and can cause more micro-trauma and tension to build up.

As the joints are not moved and stretched during this activity, any increase in tension often goes unnoticed and the condition may be allowed to build up over a long period of time. The muscles become hard and inelastic, with pain eventually developing around the outside of the elbow. Sometimes, after a gradual build-up of tension, an overload can cause a strain or rupture, with the sudden onset of acute pain. In extreme cases, the tendon may detach from the bone (avulsion), which requires prompt medical attention.

Treatment

All the forearm muscles can be treated in the supine position, with the patient's elbow resting on the couch and the wrist held gently by the

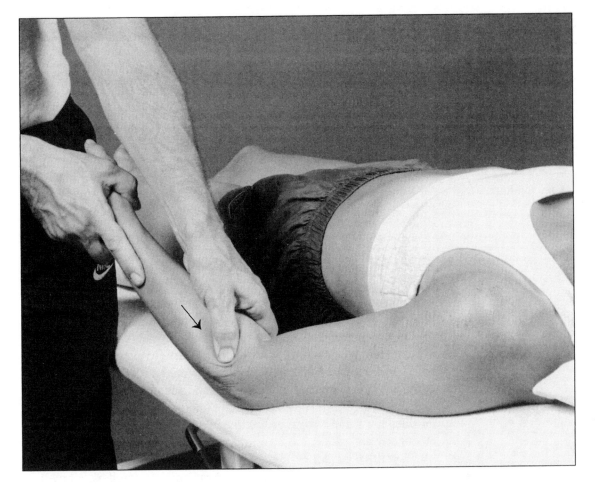

Stroking with the thumb along the forearm muscles on the radial side.

therapist in an elevated position and/or resting along the couch. By rotating the forearm from the wrist, the muscles to be treated can be turned to face whichever hand the therapist wishes to use to apply the stroke.

Particular attention should always be paid to these muscles whenever the arm is given massage, as it is better to find and treat any problem early. Everyone has some tension here and that is normal, but any excessive hardness or pain in the tissues should be treated with friction and stroking techniques. To reach the origins, the elbow should be flexed to relax the muscles so that the fingers can work deep into the joint to reach the humerus.

Stretching these muscles is very important after treatment, but should be done cautiously in the post-acute phase. Preventative treatment and advice on self-management are the best approach for people involved in activities with a high risk of 'tennis elbow'. Self-massage and stretching can easily be done several times a day if necessary.

(To stretch: the elbow must be fully extended, wrist palmar-flexed, and the forearm slightly pronated.)

Forearm (palmar side)

MUSCLE	ORIGIN	INSERTION	ACTION
Pronator teres	Above the medial epicondyle and coranoid process of ulna	Middle, lateral radius	Pronates and flexes forearm
Pronator quadratus	Palmar surface of ulna (distal quarter)	Palmar surface of radius	Pronates forearm
Common flexors	Medial epicondyle of humerus Upper and middle radius and ulna	Metacarpals, aponeurosis and phalanges	Flexes wrist, fingers and thumb

Apart from the pronator muscles that attach across the two bones, the flexor muscles run through long tendons, beneath a retinaculum across the wrist joint, and into the fingers. We require considerable strength in flexing the fingers for gripping-type actions, which should require big muscles. But to have large muscles in the hand would restrict dexterity, which is of such paramount importance in the hand. Instead, the power comes from the muscles in the forearm and is transmitted through the tendons to create strong flexion in the fingers. (Although some of these muscles have their origin at the humerus, they have minimal effect on elbow movement.)

Repetitive activities involving gripping can lead to tension and pain developing in these upper forearm muscles ('golfer's elbow'). If wrist movements are also involved, inflammation can occur at the retinaculum, due to rubbing or compression (carpal tunnel syndrome).

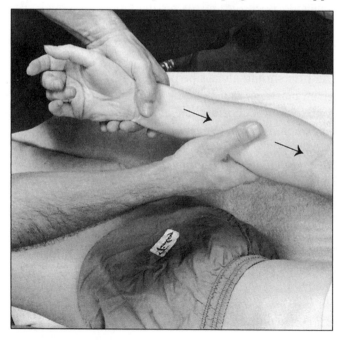

Stroking with the thumb along the muscles on the palmar side.

Treatment
Turning the palmar side up, deep strokes can be applied from the wrist to the elbow along these muscles. Friction around the origins at the inner crease of the elbow should not be too deep, because the brachial artery and vein run superficially through this area. Friction can be applied around the retinaculum to help the tendons glide smoothly. When stretching these muscles after treatment, the fingers must be included in the movement.

'Golfer's elbow' (medial epicondylitis)

This is a similar condition to 'tennis elbow' but at the medial epicondyle, caused by strain or tension in these flexor muscles. It should be treated in the same manner as 'tennis elbow'.

Carpal tunnel syndrome

The retinaculum across the palmar side of the wrist pulls the outer bones towards each other so that a tunnel is created, through which the tendons and median nerve pass. Constant pressure or impact can cause micro-trauma and scar tissue to develop and can generally congest the tunnel. This can have a rubbing or constricting effect on these tissues, which may cause further inflammation. Where the tendons are affected there may be pain and dysfunction in the hand and fingers, and if the nerve becomes tethered in the tunnel, then the symptoms may be numbness and tingling in the fingers.

Deep friction around the carpal tunnel is a good preventative measure for people who may be at risk due to their sport or occupation. The condition can develop over a long period before painful symptoms appear, by which time the congestion may be considerable. Deep friction may have some beneficial effect but at best will be very slow. Too much friction at any one time could cause inflammation, which might add to the problem. Medical and surgical procedures can often provide a quicker and more effective result.

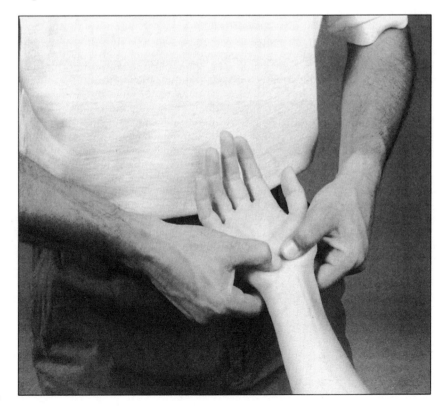

Friction with the thumbs around the carpal tunnel.

Forearm (dorsal side)

MUSCLE	ORIGIN	INSERTION	ACTION
Supinator	Lateral epicondyle and ulnar crest	Lateral surface of upper radius	Supinates forearm
Abductor pollicis longus	Dorsal surface of radius and ulna	Phalanges of thumb	Extends and abducts thumb
Extensor pollicis brevis			
Extensor pollicis longus			

These are the smallest of the muscle groups of the forearm and also have long tendons, which pass under a retinaculum before attaching to the fingers. The movements they create rarely require much force, and these muscles are not naturally very strong. But in the use of keyboards, for example, they are under constant strain, lifting and holding the hands and fingers above the keys. In this situation they can become chronically tense, and due to the tendons rubbing against the retinaculum these can become inflamed (tenosynovitis). Painful symptoms can occur anywhere along the dorsal forearm or wrist and can become very debilitating (this is a common symptom in Repetitive Strain Injury – RSI).

Treatment

Treatment can be given with the forearm rotated so that the dorsal side is uppermost. The muscles are then treated in the same manner as the muscles on the palmar side.

Below (left): Stroking with the thumb along the muscles on the dorsal side.

Below (right): Friction to the back of the wrist with the thumbs.

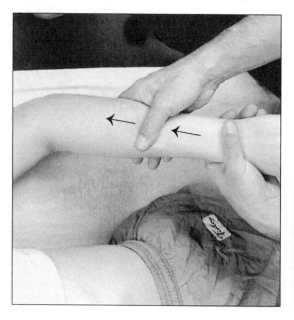

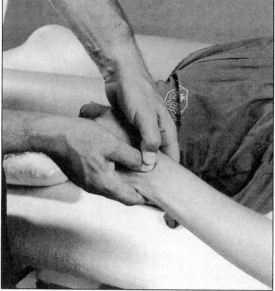

Muscles of the palm

MUSCLE	ORIGIN	INSERTION	ACTION
(Thenar eminence) Pollicis muscles	Lateral 3 metacarpals and flexor retinaculum	Metacarpal and proximal phalanx (thumb)	All inward movements of thumb
(Hypothenar eminence) Digit minimi	Medial 2 metacarpals and flexor retinaculum	Metacarpal and proximal phalanx (5th finger)	All inward movement of the ulnar border of hand

There are numerous small muscles in the hand that move the individual finger joints. The largest and most powerful of these are grouped together to form the area of the thenar eminence. Each small muscle moves the thumb in a slightly different direction, and repetitive use can lead to tension developing in particular compartments. Impact damage is also fairly common in falls, etc. The hypothenar eminence is composed of a similar but smaller group of muscles on the ulnar side of the palm.

Treatment

Although these muscles are relatively small compared to others in the body, they need to be very carefully and thoroughly palpated, because of the intricate movements they are capable of performing. Tight areas are normally found around the origins just below the wrist, but can also be found elsewhere in the group. Friction is the main treatment technique to use on any small areas of tension that may be found.

These muscles often become weak following injury, and strengthening exercises are necessary to restore normal function. These need to be done through the full range of movement and in all directions.

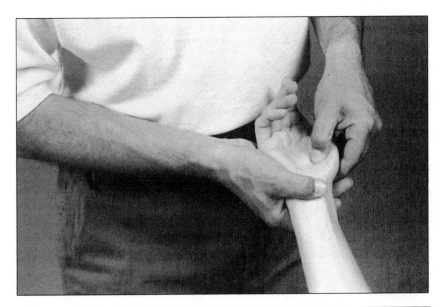

Friction to the muscles of the palm using the thumbs.

Leg (posterior)

Hip extensors (gluteals)

MUSCLE	ORIGIN	INSERTION	ACTION
Gluteus maximus	Medial iliac crest and sacrum	Iliotibial band and gluteal tuberosity of femur	Extends and outwardly rotates hip
Gluteus medius	Upper surface of ilium	Great trochanter of femur	Anterior: flexes and inwardly rotates hip Posterior: abducts and outwardly rotates hip
Gluteus minimus	Lower surface of ilium		Abducts and inwardly rotates hip

As well as extending the hip, these powerful muscles can also act in the other direction by raising the trunk from a forward-bending position. Due to the particular location of the attachments of the individual muscles, each also assists movement in other directions. The *gluteus maximus* is the largest and most powerful of these muscles and lies superficially. It provides the main force of hip extension, with the two other muscles being involved more in control and stability of the movement. Together they play a major role in all running, jumping, climbing and standing activities, and they often become strained or tight as a result of overload or repetitive use. Acute injury tends to occur towards the smaller muscle insertions.

Tension in these muscles could also be the symptom of a problem in the sacroiliac joint, especially if symptoms are found in the gluteus medius on only one side. So friction should always be applied around this joint area as well when treating these muscles. If the tension does not improve despite good massage treatment, the patient should be referred for osteopathic assessment.

Bio-mechanical faults, such as leg-length discrepancy, a turned-out leg or excessive pronation, can lead to muscular imbalance in this group. Sometimes the cause of the problem cannot be corrected, so regular massage and/or stretching and strengthening exercises can be used to prevent the symptomatic problems.

The gluteus maximus rarely gets strained, because the smaller muscles are more likely to tear first under extreme effort. Chronic tension can develop, especially if the muscle is working from an extended position, with the hip very flexed, as in climbing activities. Micro-trauma and tension usually build up around the origin at the iliac crest.

The *gluteus medius* is divided into two halves: the anterior half acts in the direction of flexion and inward rotation, while the posterior half acts to abduct and outwardly rotate. Both parts work together, one side contracting eccentrically while the other contracts concentrically. In this way the gluteus medius controls the lateral stability of the hip joint through both flexion and extension. It is therefore under constant use during running-type activities and is commonly found to be the most tense muscle of the group. Micro-trauma tends to occur at both attachments and also in the belly of the muscle. Painful symptoms sometimes refer into the hamstrings.

The *gluteus minimus* lies beneath the medius, and it is rarely possible to distinguish between the two with palpation. They are therefore treated together.

Treatment
In the prone position, deep thorough treatment needs to be given using all the massage techniques. Special attention should be paid along the iliac crest and sacral border, where tight areas are commonly found.

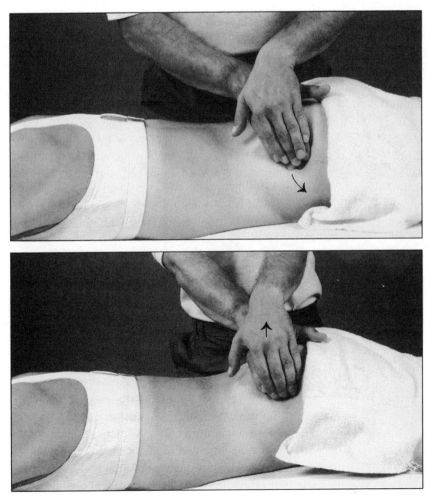

Deep stroking with the fingers through the gluteal muscles, from the iliac crest to the great trochanter.

With fingers in a hooked position, very deep strokes and friction can be applied through the gluteal muscles by pulling back across the body.

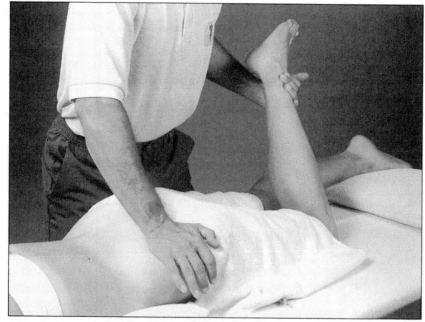

Right and below: Deep pressure can be applied in various positions into the gluteal muscles, with a stroking movement being created by rotating the hip, by rocking the lower leg back and forth.

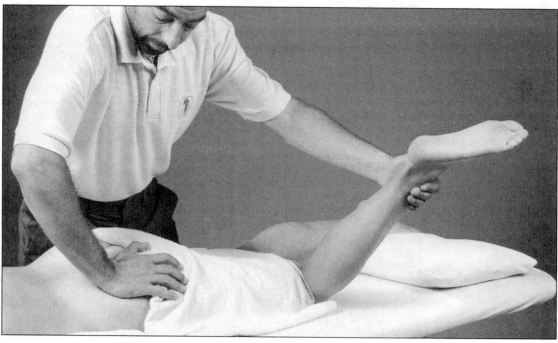

Friction should be applied slowly as it can cause considerable pain, and NMT (see Chapter 14) works very well here.

Once the maximus muscle relaxes and softens, deep long strokes can be performed through the medius muscle, working slowly from the iliac crest through to the great trochanter. As this area softens, local tight spots become more apparent and deep friction, often done with the elbow, can be applied to good effect.

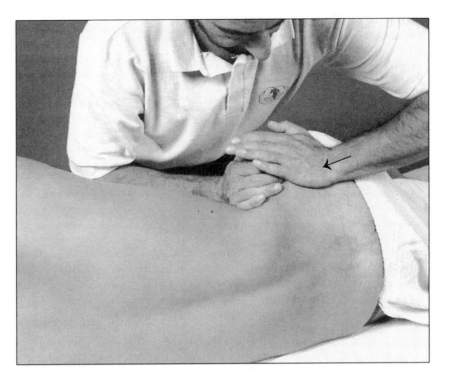

With one hand above the iliac crest, the heel of the other hand can push towards it to apply deep pressure into the gluteal muscles.

Very deep transverse strokes can be applied by leaning across the patient to treat the muscles on the other side. The therapist's body weight (with the arms straight) can be used to push the stroke from the sacrum round to the great trochanter, and with the fingers curled into the tissues, the return stroke can pull back from the tensor fascia lata. This is the clearest way of feeling tight bands in the muscle, which can then be treated with friction and longitudinal strokes (see p.163).

The gluteals can also be treated in the side-lying, hip-flexed position, which puts a slight stretch on the muscles and makes the techniques more powerful. It also changes the alignment of the tissues, and by working from both sides of the couch, different angles and directions can be used to explore and treat the area fully. Elbow techniques are very powerful in this position but should be done with care.

In the prone position there is a deep general technique that can treat the whole group, including the piriformis. The therapist applies heavy pressure through the heel of the palm into the centre of the muscle area. With the other hand, the patient's ankle can be held in an elevated position, so that the knee is flexed. This is then used as a lever to rock the leg back and forth (sideways). This moves the muscles, stretching and shortening them, which has a stroking effect with the passive pressure. By moving the pressure into different areas within the group it is possible to assess all the muscles as they move, and to apply deeper, more focused pressure through the thumb (or elbow) where local problems are felt. Friction is created by moving the tissues rather than the therapist's digit (see p.164).

Outward hip rotators			
MUSCLE	ORIGIN	INSERTION	ACTION
Piriformis	Anterior surface of sacrum	Great trochanter of femur	Outwardly rotates and abducts hip
Obturator internus	Ilium, ischium and pubis		
Obturator externus	Lower surface of ilium		Outwardly rotates and adducts hip
Quadratus femoris	Ischial tuberosity	Posterior, inferior to great trochanter	

These are deep muscles in the lower hip area, which outwardly rotate the leg, but since there are few activities in life that require this movement to be performed with any great force, these muscles are more involved in controlling movement, by preventing excessive inward rotation. This requires eccentric contraction, which is more strenuous on the muscles, and as they only go through a very small range of movement, tension can often increase with repetitive use. Bio-mechanical faults from the leg can create a greater demand for control by these muscles, which can also add to the stress.

Dance and gymnastic-type activities do require forced external rotation, and these muscles must be trained specifically over a long period of time, and from an early age, to enable them to cope with such demands. Over-use injury and trauma can occur in these activities.

The sciatic nerve (which can be as thick as a finger in this area) passes in between these muscles, and in some people actually passes through the *piriformis*. Excessive muscle tension can impinge on the nerve and lead to sciatic pain down the leg. Sometimes a seemingly serious condition of 'sciatica' can be effectively treated by the simple use of massage to release the muscles and break adhesions that may be tethering the nerve.

Painful trigger-points are often found in the piriformis which can affect the whole area. It is therefore perhaps the most important muscle of the hip, in terms of treatment. It should be returned to several times during a session so that it can be worked on more deeply and thoroughly each time.

Treatment

Because patients normally wear some clothing around this part of the body, for practical purposes the therapist usually treats the piriformis along with the gluteals, and the other muscles along with the hamstrings.

When treating the piriformis in the prone position, the true origin lies beneath the sacrum and can only be reached as it comes out from

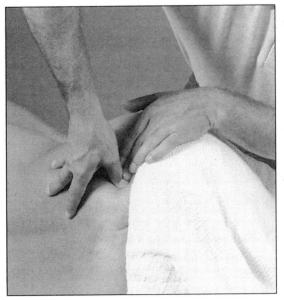

In a side-lying, hip-flexed position, deep friction with the thumb can be applied into the origin of the piriformis, deep behind the sacrum bone.

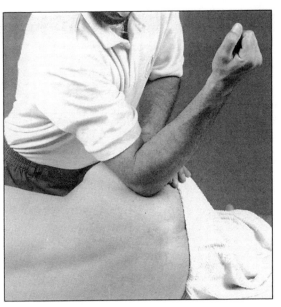

Deep friction into the piriformis muscle with the elbow.

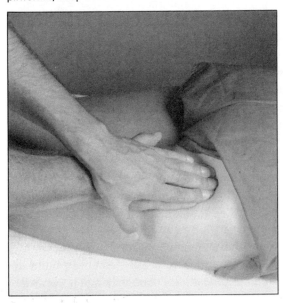

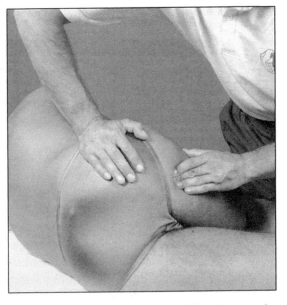

Above (left): Deep stroking and friction with the fingers into the outward hip rotators.

Above (right): In a side-lying, hip-flexed position, the outward hip rotators can be treated with friction using the fingers.

behind the lateral border. From here, deep stroking and friction can be used to good effect all the way to the insertion. In the side-lying, hip-flexed position, deep friction can be applied in a downward direction behind the sacrum to reach the origin more easily.

The three other muscles can be reached from the top of the hamstrings, and fill a hollow space that can be felt between the ischium and the great trochanter. All stroking and friction techniques can be used in the prone position. The side-lying, hip-flexed position is good for deeper friction around the origins at the ischium.

Hamstrings			
MUSCLE	ORIGIN	INSERTION	ACTION
Biceps femoris	Ischial tuberosity	Lateral tibial condyle and lateral head of fibula	Primary: flexes knee Secondary: extends hip
Semimembranosus		Medial tibial condyle	Also: stabilizes knee when extended and slight rotation when flexed
Semitendinosus			

The hamstring muscles form the area at the back of the thigh. As well as flexion, the hamstrings help stabilize the knee joint when it is in extension. They are also involved in the slight rotation of the lower leg when the knee is flexed, which is very significant in the bio-mechanics of walking and running. It is therefore important to assess and treat the hamstrings with all cases of knee, lower leg or foot problems.

Acute strains are fairly common through over-use or over-stretching in many sports, especially those involving powerful knee flexion, like sprinting. Accidental injury is also fairly common if the leading leg slips forward, forcing a sudden eccentric contraction of the muscles in an effort to prevent a fall.

Injury may occur anywhere along the belly of the muscles as well as at the attachments. Strains are more likely towards the origins, along the ischial tuberosity, in activities involving strong contraction when the hip is flexed and the hamstring muscles extended, like jumping or climbing activities. Chronic over-use injuries are more common at the distal muscle/tendon junctions and towards attachments at the back of the knee, where micro-trauma often occurs and fibrosis builds up.

The muscles are frequently found to be quite tight, which is usually due to a poorly balanced training programme. Sportsmen often put more effort into building strength and flexibility in the quadriceps and pay less attention to their hamstrings. In this situation they can easily suffer from over-use, and micro-trauma can develop. This is often found at a very deep level in the muscle, and fibrous adhesions can build up and go unnoticed and untreated, unless very deep massage is applied.

Tension or pain in the hamstrings could also be associated with lower back problems. The hips and lower back should always be treated along with the hamstrings, particularly if there has been no obvious cause for an apparent leg injury. In mild cases of 'sciatica' the symptoms are sometimes only felt in the hamstrings of one leg. Initially this may appear, to the patient, to be a muscle problem, but treating the muscle will achieve very little. If the sciatic nerve is the cause of the problem, a passive straight leg-raise stretch will be severely limited by pain, but the therapist will not feel any muscular resistance at this point.

Treatment

The hamstrings are a very large muscle group, and in the case of a powerful athlete there could be several inches of tissue between the outer surface of the leg and the bone. After softening the area superficially with general techniques, a combination of deep work with transverse strokes, friction and longitudinal strokes should be used. This should help release adhered fibres.

To reach the very deepest tissues, the patient can be placed in a half side-lying position with the hip and knee of the injured leg flexed. To treat the medial side, the injured leg should be the lower; for the lateral side, it should be the overlying leg. This position enables deep friction

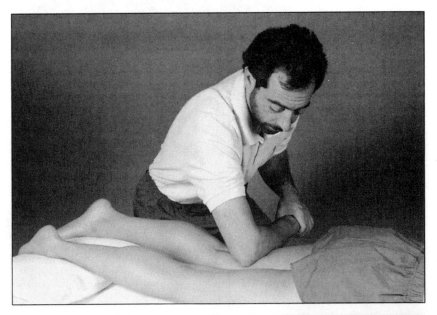

Deep stroking with the forearm through the hamstring muscles.

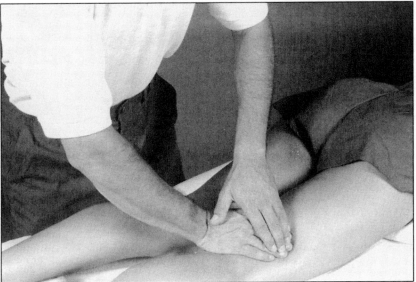

Friction with the fingers into the biceps femoris tendon.

Right: Friction with the thumbs, working in from the medial border to reach the deep fibres of the hamstrings close to the bone.

Below (left): In a half-side-lying position, one hand can lift the hamstring muscles and the fingers of the other hand can apply friction from the lateral border into the deep fibres close to the bone.

Below (right): In a half-side-lying position with the hip flexed, friction can be applied with the fingers into the hamstring origins at the ischial tuberosity.

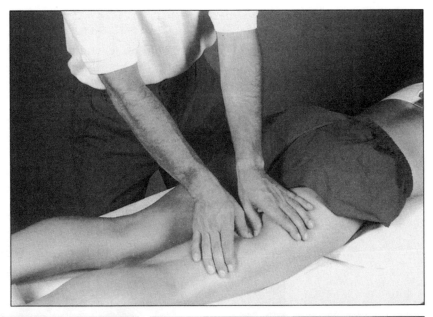

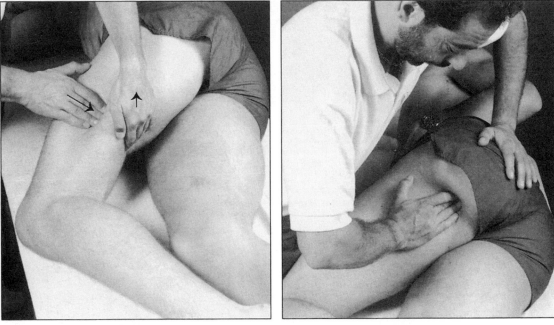

to be applied from the side of the leg, one way, deep into the muscle belly, or the other way into the tissues next to the bone. In extreme chronic cases this may require the use of the elbow.

To reach the origins at the ischial tuberosity, the half side-lying position with the hip flexed also allows very good access. One hand can be placed above the iliac crest to fix the position and provide an anchor to push against. The thumb or fingers of the other hand can then be used to apply friction. In the prone position it is necessary to curl the fingers deep under, then up and behind the gluteus maximus to reach it.

Popliteus			
MUSCLE	ORIGIN	INSERTION	ACTION
Popliteus	Posterior, lateral femoral condyle and posterior lateral meniscus	Superior, posterior tibia	Flexes knee

The popliteus is a small, deep muscle that runs diagonally across the back of the knee and is the only muscle to flex this joint alone It stabilizes the lateral side of the joint and draws the meniscus back when the knee is flexed. It can become tense, particularly if there are problems in adjacent muscles, or with lateral meniscal injuries. Problems are also more likely to occur in people with hyper-extension at the knee, which stretches the muscle. Swelling in this area, however, could be due to a 'baker's cyst' (a swelling of the posterior joint capsule caused, usually, by an inflamed bursa). Although uncommon, this should be considered, and referred to a medical practitioner if there is no apparent damage to other local tissues, and if there is pain on full passive flexion.

Treatment
This muscle can be palpated with the knee resting in a fairly flexed position. Gentle stroking techniques can be used, but deep friction should not be applied in this area because of the underlying blood vessels.

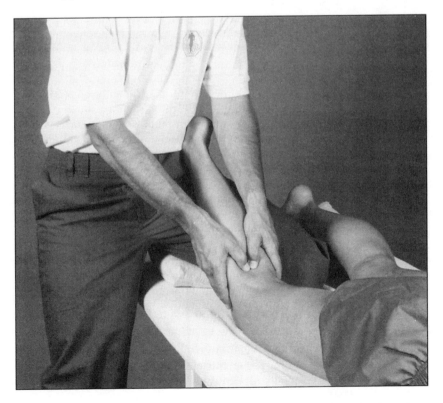

With the lower leg elevated and resting on the therapist's thigh (to flex the knee), the thumbs can be used to stroke and friction the popliteus muscle.

Plantaris			
MUSCLE	ORIGIN	INSERTION	ACTION
Plantaris	Above the lateral femoral condyle	Via a long tendon to the medial, posterior calcaneum	Flexes knee and plantaflexes foot

The plantaris muscle is not noted for its action, other than assisting the gastrocnemius in knee flexion and foot plantaflexion. However, its shape and position would suggest that it is important in co-ordinating the positioning of the knee and ankle during walking and running-type movements. It rarely suffers from major problems but can become swollen (at the back of the knee) in activities like ballet, particularly where there is hyper-extension in the knee.

Although a small muscle, it has a very long tendon passing medially between the gastrocnemius and soleus muscles before attaching to the calcaneum bone. Excessive tension along this tendon can irritate and cause inflammation where it passes under the inferior medial aspect of the gastrocnemius. Local treatment for symptomatic pain in this area will give only temporary relief if the plantaris muscle itself is not specifically treated and stretched.

Treatment
The plantaris is treated along with the other calf muscles.

Posterior compartment (lower leg)			
MUSCLE	ORIGIN	INSERTION	ACTION
Gastrocnemius	Posterior, medial and lateral femoral condyles	Via Achilles tendon to posterior calcaneum	Plantaflexes foot and flexes knee
Soleus	Upper two-thirds of posterior tibia and fibula		Plantaflexes foot

The relationship between the gastrocnemius and the soleus is important when considering sport and injury. The gastrocnemius is the main plantaflexor of the foot only when the knee is in extension, and it is assisted by the soleus. When the knee is flexed, however, the gastrocnemius is shortened and is less able to contract, so the soleus becomes the main plantaflexor. This means that there is less power when pushing off from the ground when the knee is bent, as the smaller soleus has to produce all the effort and it is therefore more vulnerable to strain in this kind of situation.

These muscles often suffer from poor training, as the sportsman may do only one type of calf stretch, so allowing tension to build up in the muscle he is neglecting. It is the soleus that is usually the more tense, and this can easily be felt by the therapist, as it will be much harder on palpation than the gastrocnemius.

Separate stretching exercises should be performed with the knee in both extension (for the gastrocnemius) *and* slight flexion (for the soleus and Achilles). Similarly, any strength training should be in both positions but with less force when the knee is bent.

Both muscles are subject to acute strain in all sports involving a strong running-type action, especially on hard surfaces or when going uphill. Chronic over-use tension can build up through micro-trauma and a large area, usually on the lateral side of the muscles, can become hard and congested before any painful symptoms appear. This can be due to bio-mechanical faults like excessive pronation, bad shoes or poor stretching. In sports such as cycling, where the soleus muscle mainly works isometrically, congestion and tightness can build up due to the static nature of the effort.

Hard running activities can make the calf muscles disproportionately strong in relation to the tibialis anterior muscle (see p.196), and this can restrict joint movement. Strengthening exercises for the anterior muscles as well as stretching (and massage) to the calf are necessary to correct this imbalance.

Treatment
General treatment for both muscles is normally done in the prone position, with the ankle slightly elevated to shorten and relax them.

The *gastrocnemius* has two bellies running side-by-side, and general massage should be applied to each separately as their conditions will be different. The lateral side is often found to be tighter and more

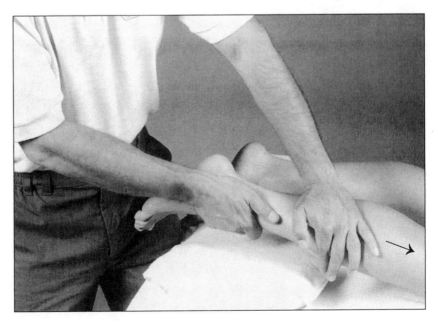

Supporting the lower leg with one hand, the palm of the other can apply strokes along the calf muscles. Pressure can be increased by pulling the lower leg up as the stroke is made.

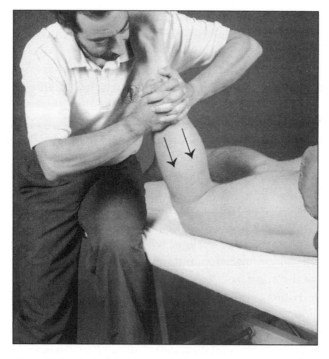

Above: With the lower leg elevated by resting the ankle on the therapist's shoulder, the heels of both hands can be used in a vice-like action as strokes are made along the calf muscles.

Right: In a side-lying position, deep stroking and friction can be applied into the deep fibres of the lateral soleus and gastrocnemius muscles.

congested, as many running and side-stepping activities put more force through this side. Long strokes and friction should be applied between the two bellies to release any adhesions and stimulate the circulation there. Transverse strokes should be applied from this central groove through either side of the muscle. To reach the origins at the femoral condyles, the therapist should flex the patient's knee so that the palpating fingers can work through shortened and relaxed tissues.

The *soleus* is a smaller, flatter muscle, which lies partly beneath the gastrocnemius and commonly tends to be tighter. The principal way to treat it is with deep stroking, usually with the thumb, working up the muscle from either side of the Achilles tendon. It is often more comfortable for the therapist to kneel with one leg on the couch and rest the patient's lower leg over it.

To release tension in the soleus it is often good to apply deep stroking along this muscle while it is fixed in a stretched position. This can be done (prone) by abducting the leg slightly so that the lower leg

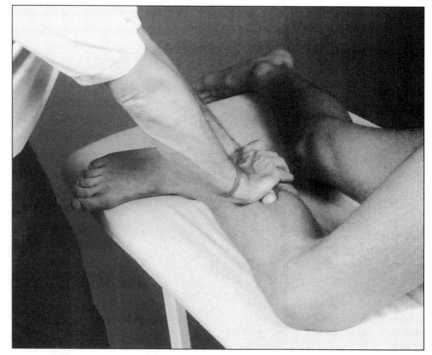

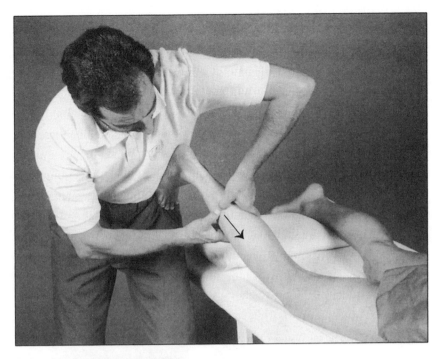

Right: With the lower leg elevated and the foot fixed in dorsiflexion against the therapist's hip to stretch the soleus muscle, deep stroking can be applied with the thumbs.

Below: With the patient's knee elevated and the therapist sitting on the foot to keep the leg stable, stroking and friction can be applied by curling the fingers into the tissues and leaning back to increase the pressure.

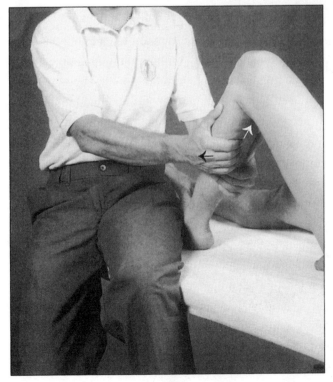

clears the side of the couch and raising it by flexing the knee. The therapist can use the side of his hip to fix the foot in dorsiflexion, which stretches the muscle and leaves both hands free to work.

Although general treatment is usually carried out in the prone position, to work on the deeper tissues a side-lying position enables friction to be applied from the side to reach the areas near the bone. It is sometimes even possible to reach the interosseous membrane (between the tibia and fibula), where scarring can restrict the movement between the bones and lead to a variety of referred problems.

The area can also be treated from the anterior side with the patient lying supine with his knee elevated and foot flat on the couch. The therapist should sit lightly on the foot to keep it still (and to warm the patient's toes) and work the muscle from behind, leaning back to apply pressure. In this position the gastrocnemius is shortened and falls away from the bone, making it easier to identify and treat the deeper tissues.

'Shin splints'

Damage can occur to the tissues along the medial tibial border with fibrous adhesion forming between the muscle and bone. This is commonly called 'shin splints', but there are in fact three possible causes of this condition:

- Scarring in the muscle fibres
- Adhesions between the muscle and bone
- Periostitis of the tibia

In chronic conditions, the border of the bone may become rough and irregular due to scarring and this can encourage further damage.

Periostitis is the least common of the three types of 'shin splints' and, even in the acute stage, it is hard to assess whether the periosteum

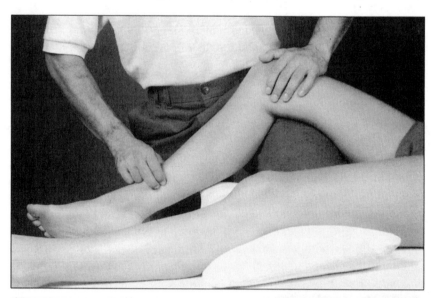

With the knee flexed and resting on the therapist's thigh, the fingers or thumb can apply deep friction and stroking along and slightly behind the medial tibial border (to treat 'shin splint' conditions).

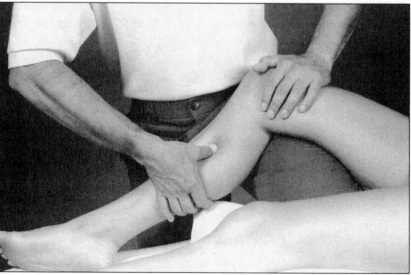

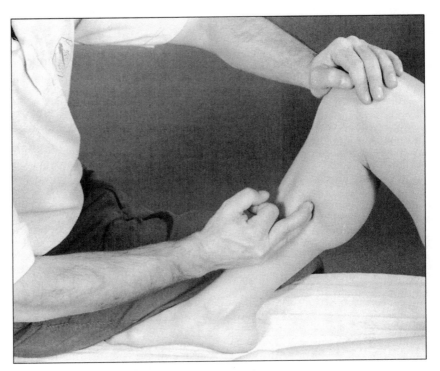

Sitting on the patient's foot and supporting the knee in an elevated position, the fingertips can curl round the bone to apply deep friction and stroking ('shin splints').

is actually involved. If it is, friction may aggravate the condition, but the other two situations respond extremely well to deep friction and stroking techniques. Initial treatment should therefore be carried out cautiously and the effects monitored, in case inflammation increases. It is also a good precaution to apply ice after this treatment.

The treatment of 'shin splints' is usually very painful and may leave residual pain for a day or two afterwards. This should be discussed first, in case it conflicts with the patient's other priorities. Self-treatment is also advisable, because a few minutes of deep friction twice a day can achieve quicker results with less pain than a long, intensive session once a week.

The *Achilles tendon* transmits the force of contraction between the gastrocnemius/soleus muscles and the calcaneum bone, so creating plantaflexion of the foot. It is of fundamental importance in nearly all activities, such as walking and running, and is a common area for acute strain and over-use. As well as the usual causes of injury, it is particularly affected by twisting and rotation movements, which are often caused by faulty bio-mechanics (pronation), poor shoes or high heel-tabs. The blood supply to this tendon is fairly good, except for an area about 2–3 inches (5–8 cm) above the calcaneus attachment, which is where injuries more commonly occur. A low level of inflammation over a period of time can result in general fibrosis building up in the area around the tendon.

The Achilles tendon is surrounded by a paratendon, which acts like a sheath, through which it runs. Over-use could result in scarring, not

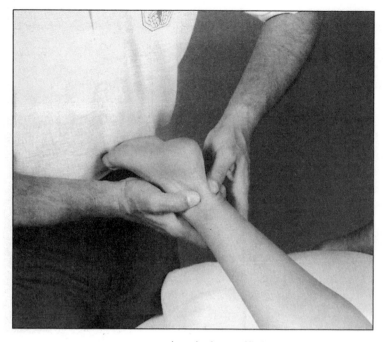

With the ankle elevated so that the therapist does not have to bend down, the thumbs can be used to apply deep stroking and friction along the Achilles tendon.

only outside the structure but also inside, between the sheath and the tendon. This can cause a creaking sensation (crepitus) to be felt when the tendon moves. Focal degeneration with scar formation within the tendon itself can also occur. Inside the sheath, friction techniques can cause further inflammation, which does not recover well due to its confinement within the sheath. So initial treatment should be given with caution and ice applied afterwards.

With the ageing process, the tendons can become drier and less pliable, as their lubrication is less efficient, so injuries are more likely and often tend to become chronic. Complete ruptures of the Achilles is not uncommon in older people, especially those involved in active sports on hard surfaces, like tennis and squash (this requires immediate medical attention and must be referred).

Irregular bony prominences (exostosis) are sometimes found along the calcaneum bone at the back of the heel, which can cause tendon inflammation. Chronic long-term inflammation near the attachment can also lead to a build-up of scar tissue. Massage will have little effect on this and may in fact aggravate it. Surgical repair is sometimes the only effective solution.

Treatment

The Achilles tendon should be treated with stroking and friction techniques, using the same positions as for the soleus. The area to the sides and behind the tendon should be treated with considerable pressure, to clear congestion and improve the circulation around it. Treatment to the tendon itself should start with only minimal pressure as the Achilles is very sensitive, and it should be increased only if the tissues appear to soften and pain reduces. Applying deep strokes up the tendon when it is in a slightly stretched position, by dorsiflexing the foot with the therapist's hip, may help release adhesions between the tendon and the inside of the sheath. Friction is also important around the calcaneum attachment, to prevent scar tissue formation, which could calcify and turn into bony prominences.

Application of ice following friction of the Achilles tendon is a good precautionary measure, as treatment may cause inflammation.

Deep posterior compartment (lower leg)			
MUSCLE	ORIGIN	INSERTION	ACTION
Tibialis posterior	Upper half of tibia and fibula and interosseous membrane	Plantar side of tarsals and metatarsals	Plantaflexes and inverts foot
Flexor digitorum longus		Distal phalanx of 4 outer toes	Plantaflexes foot and toes. Inverts foot
Flexor hallucis longus		Distal phalanx of big toe	Plantaflexes foot and big toe. Inverts foot

The muscles of the deep posterior compartment are difficult to palpate but can be reached just behind the tibia, if the superficial muscles are sufficiently relaxed. The tendons can be felt more easily as they pass around the medial malleolus, where they can become inflamed due to rubbing (tarsal tunnel syndrome). They run into the sole of the foot, but only the flexor digitorum longus tendon can be felt as it emerges from beneath the plantar muscles and attaches to the big toe. Chronic tension here can result in a painful thickening along the tendon, which can affect the mechanics of the foot and lead to other lower leg symptoms.

These muscles flex the toes and are important when springing from the ground, and they help control all movements of the foot. Over-use problems can develop due to heavy repetitive footwork, particularly on hard or uneven surfaces. Bio-mechanical faults, like excessive pronation/supination or excessive inward/outward foot rotation, as well as structural faults, like a low foot arch, are also likely to encourage injury. Secondary tension usually develops in association with ankle injuries, especially sprains.

Treatment

These muscles are difficult to treat because of their location. After the superficial muscles have been relaxed, the best access is usually achieved with the patient in the supine position, with the knee elevated and the foot flat on the couch. In this way it is easier to feel the deep posterior compartment muscles, which remain fairly stretched while the other calf muscles are shortened and relaxed. The therapist should sit slightly on the foot and work around the leg, and pull back to stroke and friction the deep tissues between the muscle and the bone running up from the ankle.

This is also a comfortable position for applying friction to the tendons around the medial malleolus. The muscles can also be treated in the prone position, with the lower leg slightly elevated and supported. Deep strokes and friction need to be applied from the side to reach the deep tissues.

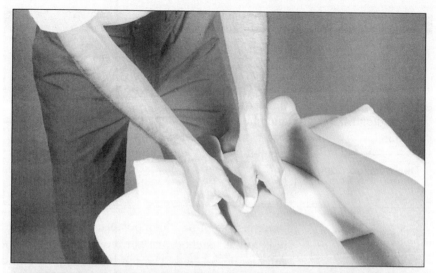

Deep friction can be applied with the thumbs into the deep posterior compartment by working in behind the lateral side of the Achilles tendon.

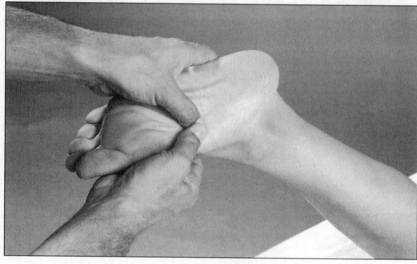

The flexor hallucis longus tendon runs through the sole of the foot to the big toe and must be treated along with the muscles of the deep posterior compartment. Here, friction and stroking with the thumbs.

The long tendon leading to the big toe responds well to friction but treatment is painful. The patient should self-treat the area, as a few minutes' daily treatment can achieve the best results.

It is very important to stretch these tissues after treatment. To do this effectively the foot must be fixed in a strongly dorsiflexed position, to pre-stretch the tissues before increasing the stretch with the toes.

Compartment syndrome (see also p.91)
This can occur in any of the muscle compartments of the lower leg, but it is most problematic when it occurs in the deep posterior compartment. Because of its depth, it cannot be reached with superficial techniques, and as deep friction may aggravate a compartment syndrome it should be treated with caution. If the condition fails to improve after one or two sessions, the patient should be referred for a medical assessment.

Plantar muscles (foot)

MUSCLE	ORIGIN	INSERTION	ACTION
Flexor digitorum brevis	Calcaneum	Middle phalanges of 4 outer toes	Flexes toes
Abductor hallucis	Medial calcaneum	Metatarsal/phalangeal joint (big toe)	Abducts and flexes big toe and maintains foot arch
Flexor hallucis brevis	Lateral cuneiform and cuboid		Flexes big toe
Abductor digiti minimi	Posterior, lateral calcaneum	Phalanx of 5th toe	Abducts 5th toe

Mechanically the foot is perhaps the most complicated structure of the body, and podiatrists who specialize in treating structural disorders of the foot are often the best people to refer difficult cases to. Structural problems can cause symptoms elsewhere in the body by affecting biomechanics. Some chronic leg, hip or back conditions may recover only if foot problems are attended to first.

The foot can suffer soft tissue injuries, which can be effectively treated with massage. General preventative massage can be highly beneficial as the feet are put under great pressure in many sports and other activities but are usually neglected in terms of care and training. When injury occurs, recovery may be slow because it is difficult to give the tissues sufficient rest in the early stages.

The *plantar fascia* (or aponeurosis) is a thick, strong fascia that covers the muscles along the sole of the foot. Its fibres run from the calcaneum bone distally to the metatarsal/phalangeal joints and also transversely across these joints. It provides the tension necessary to create the longitudinal and transverse arches of the foot. Hard repetitive footwork can cause a build-up of micro-trauma, which may result in inflammation (plantar fasciitis), with symptoms usually felt near the calcaneum bone. Recovery is often slow, because any movement of the foot in the early stages can cause further irritation. Deep stroking techniques can promote recovery, but as they may also cause some inflammation this does not always achieve positive results. It is impossible to distinguish through palpation what is inflammation of the fascia and what is soft tissue damage to the underlying muscles (it can be both). The former does not respond too well to massage but the latter does.

All the main muscles in the sole of the foot work together, allowing the arches to flatten and absorb the shock when landing (working eccentrically) and to contract to give spring when pushing off. Hard effort can cause over-use injury in any of these muscles, frequently in association with plantar fasciitis. The *flexor digitorum brevis* flexes the three middle toes, and a weakness will allow the transverse arch to drop. This increases compression under the metatarsal/phalangeal joints, which may become inflamed, and can impinge the nerve, so encouraging 'Morton's neuroma'.

The big toe is of major importance in all running, walking and balancing activities. Tension through over-use can build up, which may cause a restriction in dorsiflexion, which can in turn affect the bio-mechanics of the whole leg. This can usually be felt as a thickening midway between the big toe joint and the heel. Friction to break this down is painful (with residual pain) but highly effective and it should be combined with stretching (the longitudinal arch must be stretched out first, before dorsiflexing the big toe to stretch this muscle effectively).

The *abductor digiti minimi* runs along the lateral side of the foot and abducts the little toe. It may suffer injury in conjunction with other tissues in traumatic situations, or suffer from over-use tension due to bio-mechanical faults like excessive pronation. A stress fracture of the metatarsal bone could be mistaken for a chronic muscle injury, so this should be considered if massage does not produce a good result.

Treatment

The plantar side of the foot can be treated with the patient in a prone or supine position. If the dorsal side is firmly supported, the therapist can use very deep pressure with a fist or even a knuckle to stroke and friction the plantar tissues. It does require thorough assessment because a very small area of scarring can sometimes be the source of considerable discomfort.

Below (left): Deep stroking and friction with the thumbs into the plantar muscles and fascia.

Below (right): With the hand cupped round the back of the heel and the dorsal foot supported against the therapist's forearm to prevent movement, deep stroking can be applied with the back of the fist. The movement is made mostly by extending the wrist.

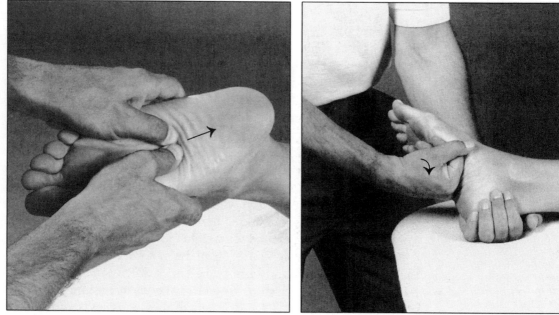

With one hand supporting the foot, the other elbow can be used to apply deep friction and stroking into the plantar muscles and fascia.

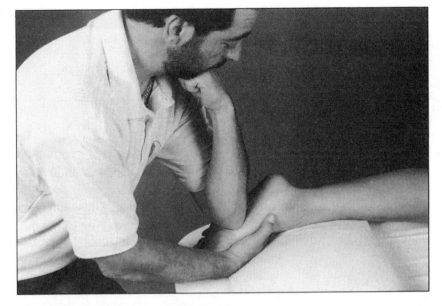

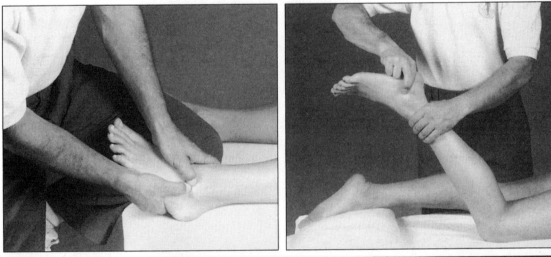

Above and right: Friction can be applied around the malleoli and the ankle joint in a variety of positions.

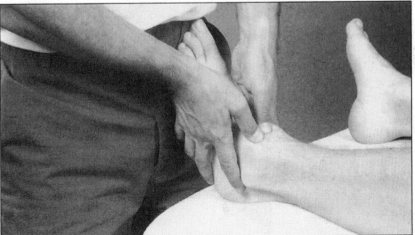

Dorsal muscles (foot)

MUSCLE	ORIGIN	INSERTION	ACTION
Extensor digitorum brevis	Calcaneum	2nd to 4th toes	Dorsiflexes toe
Extensor hallucis brevis		Big toe	Dorsiflexes big toe

The dorsal part of the foot does not contain large muscles, as the force of contraction in dorsiflexion comes through long tendons from muscles in the anterior lower leg. These long tendons run under a strong retinaculum, which runs across the top of the ankle and gives the joint the overall shape needed for its range of movement. Inflammation can occur under this retinaculum due to friction if the anterior muscles (usually the tibialis anterior) are tight. Local treatment is successful only if the associated muscle tension is also attended to.

The extensor digitorum and hallucis brevis are small muscles on the dorsal surface of the foot. They can become injured in traumatic situations, or subject to over-use strain in activities like ballet due to standing on toe points.

Pain in the dorsal surface of the foot may be due to tendonitis created by a rubbing pressure on the tendons. This is usually caused by shoe-lacing that is too tight or that comes too far up the foot. Massage to promote healing will help, but a simple remedy is to change the lacing pattern to avoid pressure on the painful area. It is sometimes advisable not to use the top lace-holes of the shoe as a preventative measure.

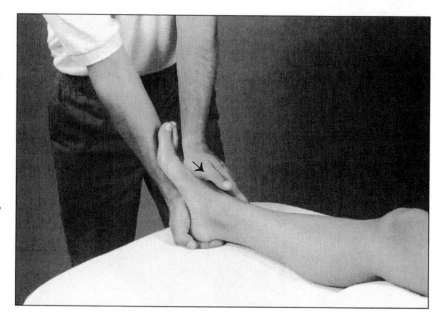

With the hand resting on the couch and cupping the back of the heel, with the sole of the foot supported against the therapist's forearm. The heel of the other hand can apply deep strokes along the dorsal surface of the foot.

Ligaments

The bones of the foot are bound together by a complex network of ligaments. These can become sprained as a result of traumatic foot or ankle injuries, which can lead to adhesions and poor function in the foot. Friction should be applied thoroughly between the bones wherever scar tissue is identified. This should be followed by general mobilization, by gently moving and twisting the foot in all directions, within a pain-free range.

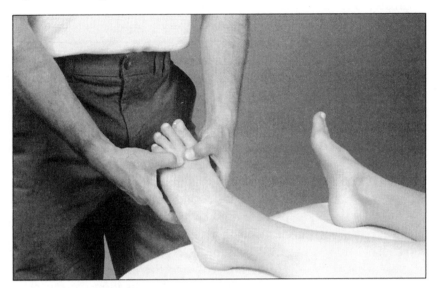

Friction can be applied with both thumbs around the ligaments and bones of the forefoot.

'Morton's neuroma'

Pain and numbness in the middle toes may be due to 'Morton's neuroma', caused by a dropping of the transverse arch between the metatarsal/phalangeal joints, which puts pressure on the plantar digital nerves. Visible signs of this may be hard skin under these central joints, the dorsal tendons appearing very prominent, and increased pain when pressing between the joints. It may be corrected by strengthening the plantar muscle, which gives support to the arch. This can be done by picking up a small object with the middle toes.

By the time this condition causes painful symptoms it has usually been developing over a very long period, and although strengthening exercises can work, results may be slow. Modern surgical methods can sometimes be the best answer in acute cases. Friction can ease pressure on the nerves, but any symptom relief will probably be only temporary if the arch remains dropped.

Bursitis

Around all the joints of the foot are numerous fat pads or bursae. These can become inflamed (bruised) in activities that involve heavy landing on hard surfaces. Although massage is helpful, a short rest period is normally the most effective solution.

Leg (anterior)

Hip flexors			
MUSCLE	ORIGIN	INSERTION	ACTION
Psoas major and minor	T12 to L4/5	Lesser trochanter of femur	Flexes hip Also: assists side-bending and inward rotation of thigh
Iliacus	Anterior, inferior iliac spine		

These are very powerful muscles, which flex the hip, and when the leg is fixed they also work the other way to flex the trunk forward. They are at the centre of the body, connecting the upper and lower halves, and have a far greater significance than their voluntary movements would suggest.

Lumbar vertebral injury, especially to the discs, often causes these muscles to go into a protective spasm to stop any movement that would increase the damage. If this happens bilaterally, the patient is unable to straighten up; if unilaterally, there will be a more twisted fixation. Chronic back conditions often result in some tightening or weakening of these muscles as they adapt to the dysfunction. Postural imbalances, particularly a forward-tilting pelvis, always involve the iliopsoas.

Pain is rarely felt in the actual muscle, and minor dysfunction may not be noticeable to the patient either. But the therapist should consider the involvement of the iliopsoas muscles whenever there is lower back or hip pain.

Acute strain is uncommon, because the rectus femoris is more likely to tear first, but if it does occur it is more probable towards the insertion, which is subjected to the greatest force. Over-use tension can develop in activities requiring repetitive and/or powerful hip flexion, especially if medial leg rotation and lateral trunk-bending are also involved. Inactivity, especially in a shortened position like sitting, can cause weakness, which increases its risk of injury and can also lead to back problems.

Treatment
The hip flexors are very difficult muscles to treat due to their deep location, starting at the anterior lumbar spine and running through the abdomen and hip areas. The iliacus is impossible to reach with palpation and can only be treated with stretching techniques. The psoas is just palpable through the side of the lower abdomen.

Long strokes can be applied to the lower part of the muscle with the patient in a side-lying position (with the injured side up). The hip of the upper leg should be flexed, with the inside of the knee resting on the couch. The therapist should stand facing the back of the patient and place one hand on the hip, just below the iliac crest, to support the stroke. The fingers of the other hand can then apply deep strokes and

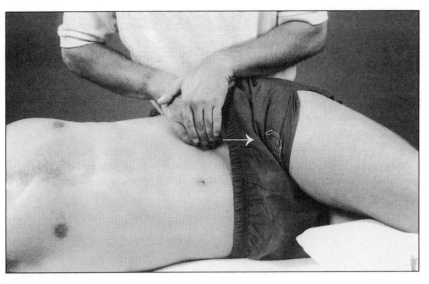

With the patient in a side-lying, hip-flexed position, the therapist should stand behind him and, leaning over, should use his hands to apply deep strokes along the lower part of the iliopsoas (hip flexor) muscles down towards the lesser trochanter.

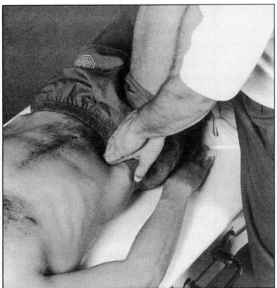

In the supine position with the hip flexed and supported passively (foot on the couch), deep pressure can slowly be applied through the lateral abdominal area into the iliopsoas muscle (contraindications for abdomen massage apply).

friction through the side of the abdomen and down towards the lesser trochanter.

Treatment can also be given in the supine position, but the patient's neck and upper back, as well as the knees, must be well elevated, and the foot flat on the couch. This shortens and relaxes the muscles of the abdomen as well as the iliopsoas. The point where pressure should be applied is on the level of the superior anterior iliac crest, halfway between it and the centre line of the body (this is about 2 inches/5 cm out and 2 inches/5 cm down from the umbilicus). Pressure needs to be extremely deep and the abdomen muscles may contract to resist this, so it must be applied very slowly. This can also be helped by increasing the pressure in stages as the patient exhales, after taking a deep breath in. When the muscle is reached, very slow friction can be applied.

As so little of the muscle can be reached, palpation may not identify a problem. The whole muscle can be tested by holding a deep passive pressure, and then the patient should attempt to lift his foot off the couch (which contracts the iliopsoas). Even though there may be minimal discomfort with just the pressure, if the muscle is tense or injured there will be a very sharp pain, which often makes it impossible to lift the leg. Both sides should be tested for comparison, especially when considering back problems.

Stretching techniques often form a major part of the treatment of these muscles, and the MET methods (see Chapter 14) are extremely effective.

Quadriceps

MUSCLE	ORIGIN	INSERTION	ACTION
Rectus femoris (RF)	Anterior, inferior iliac spine	Via patella and infrapatella tendon to tibial tuberosity	Flexes hip and extends knee
Vastas lateralis	Femur	Patellar border and patellar ligament to tibial tuberosity	Extends knee
Vastas intermedialis			
Vastas medialis			

The three vastas muscles extend the knee (one-joint muscles) and the rectus femoris (RF) extends the knee and also flexes the hip (two-joints). The difference is so significant that it is misleading commonly to refer to them as 'quadriceps' as if they all act in the same way.

The RF is a postural muscle, which works constantly with other flexor and extensor postural muscles, and it is directly associated with the tilt of the pelvis. It is therefore under different stresses and so can develop problems quite independently of the vastas muscles.

Injuries in sport are common because poor training methods may not equally work these different muscles. Stretching and strengthening exercises for the quadriceps normally involve flexing and extending the knee. But if these are done while the hip is in flexion (even slightly), then the RF is shortened and will be unaffected by the exercise.

Excessive tension is common in the RF and can cause a tighter pull over the anterior structures of the knee. This can lead to adhesions forming above the superior patella, inflammation of the infrapatellar bursae and/or tendon, or inflammation under the patella.

Imbalance can also occur between the three vastas muscles, due to uneven development of strength and flexibility. The vastas medialis is particularly important, as its distal fibres run transversely and so control the lateral position (tracking) of the patella as it glides up and down.

It is the imbalance of strength and/or weakness within the quadriceps group that is the most common cause of chronic knee pain. An imbalance can affect the tracking of the patella, pulling it to one side or causing it to rotate as it glides between the femoral condyles. This can cause rubbing to the articular surfaces, which may become inflamed ('runner's knee'). It may also cause micro-trauma and a build-up of scar tissue around the border of the patella.

An over-development of strength or tension in the lateral muscles can cause an outward rotation of the leg, which can affect many other areas.

The quadriceps can suffer strains in any activity involving heavy or explosive leg power. Over-use problems can develop in these muscles, as they are easy to strengthen but often inadequately stretched. Acute strains tend to occur in the more proximal parts, and over-use injuries tend to build up in the more distal parts, especially the medial patella, as well as at the origins in the hip area.

In contact sports, the quadriceps may be subjected to impact, which can cause oedema and damage in the tissues very deep near the bone. After one or two treatment sessions, and rest, painful symptoms may disappear but there can still be considerable scarring present. Without the pain, normal activity is often resumed too quickly, and these deep tissues can become permanently fibrous and adhered. Very old injuries such as these can be felt as small, hard lumps and are commonly found in the quadriceps muscles, particularly on the lateral side. If there is little or no discomfort when palpated, and there are no referred problems, these areas need not be specially treated as little will be achieved.

Treatment
Treatment of the quadriceps needs to be deep and thorough to assess all the muscles properly. Where knee problems are involved, the tissues around the patella should be palpated very deeply to identify any small areas of scarring, which can cause considerable dysfunction.

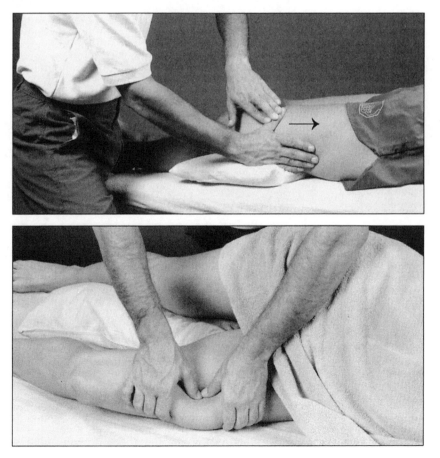

Deep stroking with the thumb along the quadriceps (vastas lateralis).

In a side-lying position, the thumbs can be used to friction in from the medial side to treat the area between the rectus femoris and the underlying muscles. (This can also be done from the lateral side when working on the other leg in this position.)

The RF needs to be singled out for a more concentrated assessment and treatment. The vastas muscles usually relax more quickly and then friction can be applied from the side, in between the RF and vastas muscles, to reach the deeper tissues. A side-lying position sometimes makes this easier.

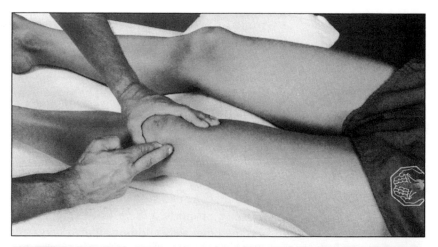

Friction around the patellar border with the fingertips.

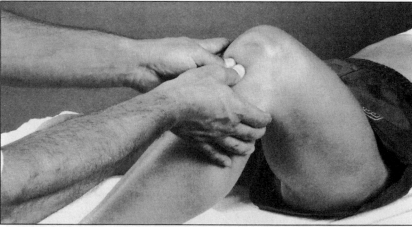

Friction with the thumbs to the infrapatellar tendon and tibial tuberosity.

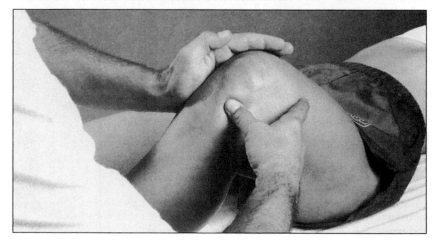

Supporting the knee on one side, the thumb of the other hand can apply friction in from the side to reach the infrapatellar bursa behind the tendon.

Sartorius			
MUSCLE	ORIGIN	INSERTION	ACTION
Sartorius	Anterior, superior iliac spine (ASIS)	Upper, medial tibial shaft	Flexes hip and knee, outwardly rotates and abducts hip

The sartorius is a very long, thin muscle running in a slight S-shape from hip to knee, and is involved more in the control of all leg movements than in the actual power. It works in association with the abdomen and quadriceps muscles but has so many functions that it is difficult to place with any particular group.

As it is seldom used to produce powerful actions, it is rarely injured, but tension can build up in association with the quadriceps. Unless it is particularly tight, it is almost impossible to feel with palpation as it blends in with the other muscles. It normally receives treatment at the same time as the thigh muscles, as it overlies them.

Treatment
To treat the sartorius specifically, the patient should be in a supine position with hip and knee flexed and outwardly rotated, and with the knee resting on the therapist's thigh. Deep stroking and friction can be applied along the muscle from the medial side of the knee, up and laterally to the anterior iliac spine.

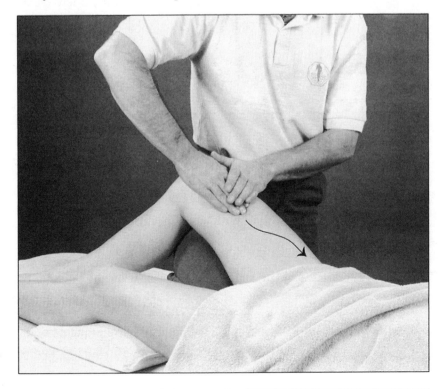

With the knee flexed, slightly abducted and supported on the therapist's thigh, long strokes can be applied with the fingers along the sartorius muscle.

Lateral hip and thigh

MUSCLE	ORIGIN	INSERTION	ACTION
Tensor fascia lata (TFL)	Anterior iliac crest	Iliotibial band	Abducts hip Also: slight flexion and inward rotation
Iliotibial band (IT)	Tensor fascia lata (muscle)	Below lateral tibial condyle	Stabilizes lateral side of knee

Leaning over the couch, the fingers can be used to apply deep stroking and friction into the tensor fascia lata muscle. Pressure can be increased by pulling back.

The *tensor fascia lata* (TFL) is a small muscle on the outside of the hip area, which is mainly involved in the lateral control and stability of the hip joint. It can become strained due to forced abduction, but this is an unusual action, so such injuries are rare. It is, however, subject to stress from other postural and bio-mechanical problems as well as from overuse. If it becomes excessively tight it may not cause pain locally but can affect the bio-mechanics of the hip and thus other areas. Endurance walking and running activities can lead to a gradual build-up of over-use tension, particularly in women, since their wider hips put more stretch on the muscle.

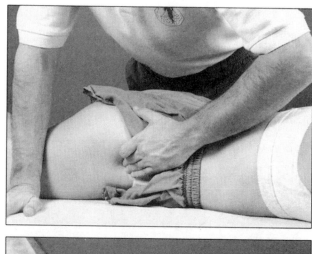

In chronic conditions, the whole muscle may feel hard, but there are usually a few local areas of greater tension within it, especially towards the origin at the iliac crest. Injury to the TFL is often mistaken for a hip problem, because painful symptoms are felt there rather than locally in the muscle. Symptoms may also be referred through the iliotibial band and cause lateral knee pain.

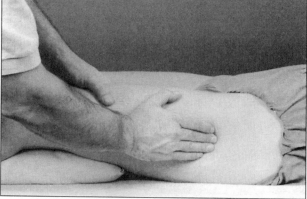

Treatment

The TFL is often neglected in general treatment as it is awkward to reach in the prone or supine positions. It should, however, receive regular treatment to release tension that may affect the function in other areas. Friction and deep longitudinal stroking from the iliac crest down to the great trochanter can be achieved with the patient in the prone position. But for deeper friction and better access, the TFL can be treated along with the hip extensors in a side-lying position.

Deep friction with the fingers into the muscle/tendon junction.

I!iotibial band (IT)   In effect, this is the tendon of the TFL muscle, connecting it to the tibia and controlling lateral knee stability, and tension can build up in association with a TFL problem. Its fascia extends over the vastas lateralis and so both are often affected together. If it becomes tight it can rub against underlying structures, usually the lateral femoral condyle, and cause inflammation there ('runner's knee'). Tension can also restrict function of the knee joint.

Treatment

Longitudinal strokes are highly effective and can be applied up the IT using the heel of the palm. More power can be gained by using the hip to press into the elbow and through to the arm and hand. Friction is also very effective, especially at the proximal muscle tendon junction. With the patient's leg extended along the couch, the therapist's fingers can often reach behind the IT at the distal end, on the lateral side of the knee, where friction can release any adhesions with deeper structures.

With one hand supporting the inside of the knee, the heel of the other hand can apply deep strokes up the iliotibial band and into the tensor fascia lata muscle. To increase pressure, the therapist can push against the elbow with his hip.

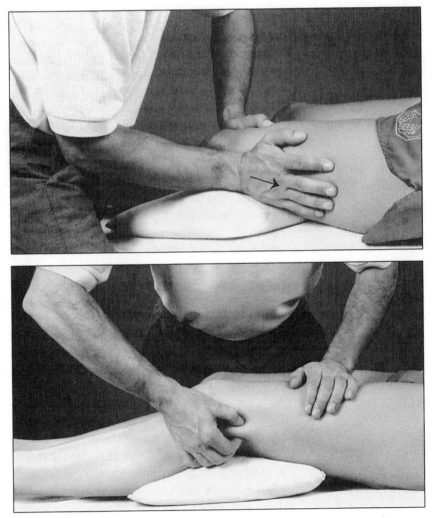

Friction can be applied to the iliotibial band, where it narrows towards its insertion, with a pinching type of action. By rocking it back and forth a friction is also applied to the tissues beneath it.

Adductors (thigh)

MUSCLE	ORIGIN	INSERTION	ACTION
Gracilis	Lower pubis	Upper, medial tibial shaft	Adducts leg, flexes knee and hip
Pectineus	Upper pubis	Linea aspera of femur and lesser trochanter	Adducts leg and outwardly rotates thigh
Adductor brevis	From pubis to ischium	Full length of medial border of femur	When leg is abducted, flexed or extended, may also inwardly rotate
Adductor longus			
Adductor magnus			
Adductor minimus			

This is a very large group made up of six muscles. As a whole they adduct the leg, but due to the specific location of the attachments, each individual muscle also has a slight involvement in other movements. The adductors can be injured in the same way as any muscle, but what determines which muscle gets strained is the secondary position or movement that also takes place. The adductor longus is the most commonly injured, as the outward rotation and abduction in which it is also involved is put under great stress in kicking activities.

Chronic tension can develop through over-use, and often goes unnoticed until an acute strain occurs somewhere in the group. As the muscles tend to spend most of their time in a shortened position, tension can easily develop in response to injury and can lead to a chronic situation. The adductors are also subject to acute strain due to over-stretching, especially in accidents like sliding falls. In activities that involve a lot of stretching, micro-trauma can occur, usually near the origin. Tissue damage here, around the pubis, is difficult to treat and often becomes chronic. Pain may be felt generally in the groin area and is often referred to as 'groin strain'.

If the adductors become weak, relative to the quadriceps, this can lead to an habitual outward rotation of the leg, which can cause many other problems. Excessive tightness can also lead to bio-mechanical problems, depending on the particular muscle affected.

Treatment
For the therapist to get good access to these muscles the patient should be supine, with the hip and knee flexed and the leg outwardly rotated. It is vital that the patient's knee is resting comfortably on cushions or the therapist's thigh, to enable the muscles to relax fully. Deep longitudinal and transverse strokes through the group should identify any tight

muscles or bands within it. These strokes should first be done using the whole hand or heel of the palm, to soften the area generally before deeper palpation and stroking are applied with the fingers. Friction should be used to release any adhered fibres, particularly in between the individual muscles. It is sometimes necessary to work right up to the ischial attachments.

Stretching is extremely important after treatment. Abduction will stretch the group in general, but to focus on a particular muscle it is necessary to add varying degrees of hip flexion and leg rotation. To add extension it is necessary to use a side-lying position or to have the patient lie slightly diagonally across the couch so that the hip and leg can hang down (and extend) off the side.

Right: With the knee flexed, slightly abducted and supported on the therapist's thigh, the heel of the hand can be used to apply deep strokes along the adductor group.

Below (left): Friction and stroking can be applied with the fingers along the individual muscles within the group.

Below (right): Individual muscles in the group that are more tense can be picked out with the fingers and friction applied to the deeper fibres in and around them.

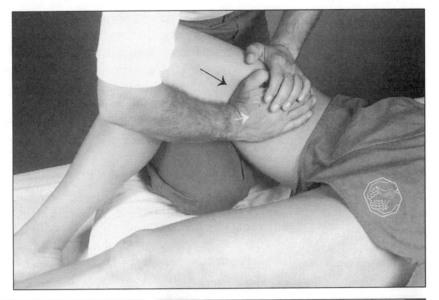

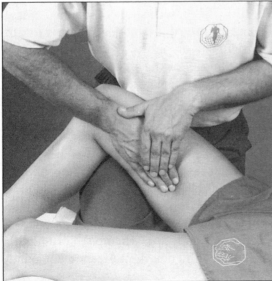

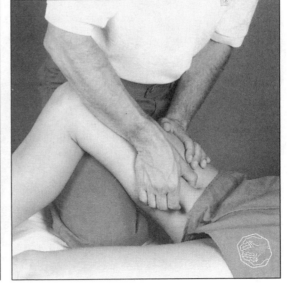

Anterior compartment (lower leg)

MUSCLE	ORIGIN	INSERTION	ACTION
Tibialis anterior	Lateral surface of tibia	Plantar surface of 1st metatarsal and medial cuneiform	Dorsiflexes foot and slight supinator
Extensor digitorum longus	Lateral tibial condyle	2nd to 5th toes	Dorsiflexes foot and toes
Extensor hallucis longus	Fibula and interosseous membrane	Distal phalanx of big toe	Extends and dorsiflexes big toe

These muscles run down the front of the shin on the lateral side of the tibia. They have long, sheathed tendons, which run under the anterior retinaculum before attaching to the toes, and so dorsiflex the foot. This is not a large movement, so these muscles work in a fairly static way. As well as contracting concentrically to lift the foot, they also have to work eccentrically to control foot-plant, stopping the forefoot from slapping down. As a result, the muscles are under constant use during all running, jumping and climbing activities and are commonly found to be tense through over-use.

If the muscles become tight, the tendons may rub against the retinaculum causing either or both to become inflamed, and a creaking (crepitus) sensation is often felt. Treating this local area of pain without attending to the tight muscle will achieve very little. The tendons can also be compressed by tight shoe-lacing, which may cause a rubbing, and inflammation, inside the sheath. This is best dealt with by rest, and by removing the external cause.

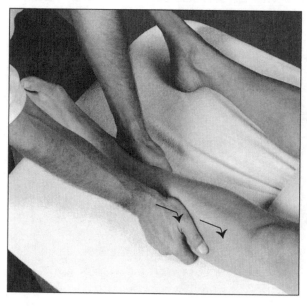

Stroking with the heel of the hand along the tibialis anterior muscle.

The muscles are contained within a fairly tight fascial sheath. A rapid increase in the size of the muscle due to strength training, or more commonly through swelling following impact trauma, can lead to compartment syndrome (see p.91).

Treatment
Deep stroking techniques up the muscles should be performed slowly, as these muscles have narrow heads and the blood cannot be forced through too quickly. Deep friction can be applied with the patient's knee elevated and his foot on the couch, and the therapist can work between the muscles to release any adhesions.

Deep stroking and friction with the thumb along the muscles of the anterior compartment.

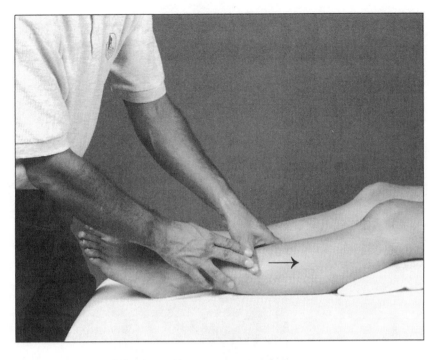

Lateral compartment (lower leg)

MUSCLE	ORIGIN	INSERTION	ACTION
Peroneus longus	Lateral aspect of fibula	Proximal, dorsal 1st metatarsal and medial cuneiform	Pronates foot and assists plantaflexion
Peroneus brevis	Lateral surface of fibula	Lateral, proximal aspect of 5th metatarsal	

These are long, thin muscles running down the lateral side, with sheathed tendons passing under the lateral malleolus and through the lateral retinaculum to the attachments in the foot. They are often found to be tight in people with excessive pronation, as this puts the muscles in a shortened position. Painful symptoms may be referred to the lateral knee area.

The tendons pass under the malleolus, where rubbing can cause inflammation. In traumatic injury these tendons can sometimes flip over the bone and remain on the wrong side of it. This causes some dysfunction but not necessarily much pain, so the patient may consider it a minor problem, but it should be referred for medical assessment.

Treatment
These muscles are treated along with the anterior compartment muscles, but with friction also applied around the malleolus.

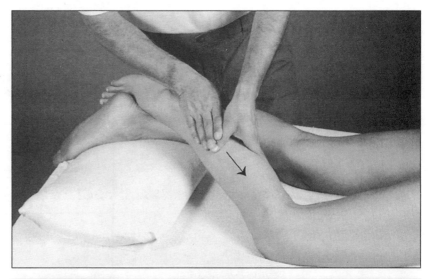

With one foot resting across the calf of the other leg, deep stroking can be applied with the thumb along the lateral compartment.

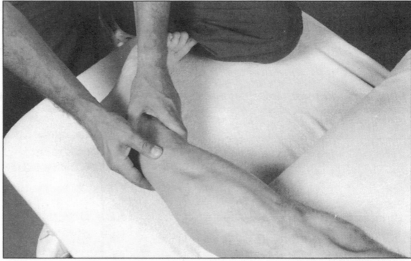

In a side-lying position, the thumb can apply friction to the peroneal tendons.

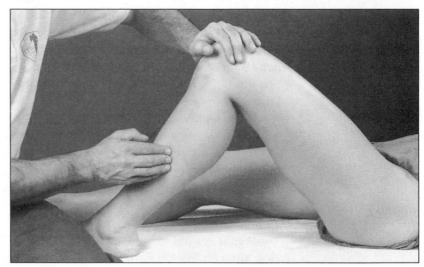

Supporting the elevated knee with one hand and sitting on the foot to stabilize the lower leg, the therapist's other hand can stroke and friction along the peroneal muscles.

14 Soft Tissue Manipulation

Neuromuscular Technique (NMT)

When musculoskeletal problems occur there is a change in the tension (tone) of the tissues concerned. This occurs naturally and is controlled automatically by the nervous system. Tension increases around a trauma (or over-use micro-trauma) to protect and contain the damage. It can also build in specific areas of tissue that are habitually held in a shortened position. Although general massage techniques can ease the tension by attending to the tissues themselves, with long-term conditions this alone may not be enough to release the hyper-tension created through the nervous system. To deal with this it is necessary to work on a neuromuscular level.

There are many therapies that are based on neuromuscular principles, but the massage therapist need not see NMT as a separate treatment method, but rather as an added ingredient to the work he already does. Indeed, the application of NMT is little more than an extension of deep friction and pressure techniques.

It has been understood throughout the long history of massage that in certain situations very deep pressure into a tender spot causes considerable pain at the time but results in a relaxation in the area afterwards. Several theories and explanations of this phenomena have emerged. It is likely that the pain factor causes a release of endorphins (a natural opiate), which suppress pain and so release tension. It is also possible that the pressure compresses the blood vessels and starves the immediate area of blood (ischaemia), and when the pressure is released the blood rushes back in. The nervous system reacts to these extreme local changes and this results in relaxation.

Through the practical application of NMT over many years it has become clear (to me) that it can best be explained in terms of the *reflex effect*: in the case of trauma, the increase in local muscle tension around the damage occurs through a natural reflex in the peripheral nervous system and is an important part of the initial healing process. However, if this situation continues for a period of time, the nervous system becomes used to holding this degree of tension and accepts it as 'normal'. This can remain the situation even if the initial trauma has long since recovered.

Where a muscle has been habitually held in a tight position due to postural, occupational or emotional factors, this degree of tension will also become accepted by the nervous system as a normal situation. Furthermore, in the long term it can naturally increase. Once local hypertension within a muscle has developed, it becomes uncomfortable to relax and stretch it, because the tight area pulls on the normal tissues around it. Instinctively the individual tends to hold the muscle even shorter to avoid discomfort, until eventually this becomes the new 'normal' level of tension.

It is important to understand that this all happens through a natural reaction (or reflex) in the nervous system, which is not consciously controlled. To treat the problem we have to bring the situation into conscious control and break the reflex pattern.

Although a patient may be aware of some discomfort or dysfunction in a muscle, he may not be aware of any particular point of actual pain. When treating the muscle, the therapist can feel any tight area and seek out the most tender spots within it. When very deep pressure is then focused on this point, it causes pain and makes the patient aware that a problem has been found. This may seem a negative course of action, but in fact the patient usually wants to find the root of the problem and is encouraged by this. Furthermore, the pain reduces as the pressure is maintained, and the patient feels this improvement take place and is further encouraged. On a psychological level, this awareness itself may in some way stimulate the recovery process.

Once the awareness of pain has been established, it is then possible to get the patient to consciously change the natural reflex pattern.

The first most instinctive reaction (or reflex action) to a painful stimulus is to avoid it by moving out of its way. But the patient resists this, because of the unique clinical situation he is in.

The next instinct is to tense the muscle to resist the pressure that is causing the pain. Instead, the patient is encouraged to relax into the pain and *not* to tense up. This is the most important factor in the technique, because it is this exact reversal that we are trying to achieve. It also requires considerable skill to make it happen properly.

Another instinct may be for the patient to concentrate on a different part of the body, such as clenching a fist or wiggling the toes, to take his mind off the pain. There is also a tendency to take very shallow breaths or even actually to hold the breath in. Encouraging the patient to breathe deeply and to focus into the point of pain can change both of these patterns, too.

By consciously focusing the patient's mind on relaxing into the pain, the nervous system is forced to suppress its normal reflex to contract. After a period of time (up to 90 seconds) the tension in the local tissues releases and the pain diminishes as relaxation occurs.

If there is an underlying cause of the problem that has not been resolved, then the tension will probably return. If it has been a long-term situation, then it could take several sessions to get a permanent result. To help maintain the improvement it is extremely important to stretch the muscle regularly for the next few days to help discourage the tissues from tensing up again and to improve functional movement and awareness.

How to apply NMT It may seem that all one has to do is find a tender spot and press into it as hard as possible for up to 90 seconds. But this would be nothing more than a brutal act which would achieve nothing. Success requires considerable subtlety.

As part of a massage treatment a particular area of tightness may be found in a muscle that feels harder and denser than would seem normal for that individual. It is important to work on this area with general

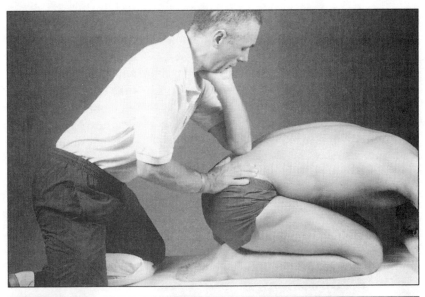

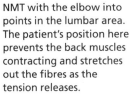

NMT with the elbow into points in the lumbar area. The patient's position here prevents the back muscles contracting and stretches out the fibres as the tension releases.

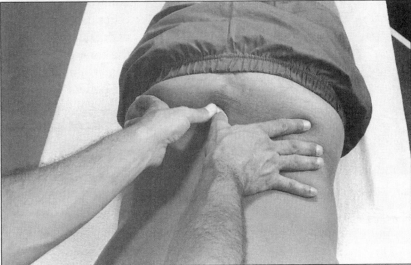

NMT with the thumbs into a point in the erector spinae attachment.

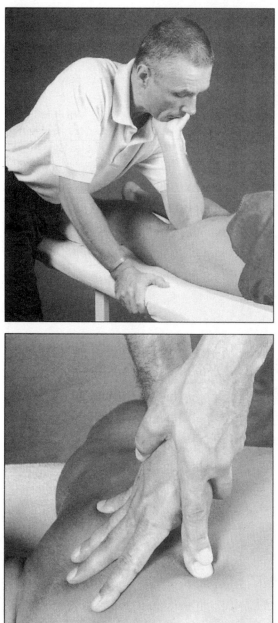

NMT with the elbow into a point in a hamstring muscle.

NMT with the tip of the thumb into a point in the rhomboid muscle.

techniques first, to warm and soften it as much as possible, and to check for contraindications. Then, with deep palpation or slow stroking, the area can be explored very thoroughly. This is usually done through a finger or thumb, but the elbow or knuckle can also be used. Within the area there may be one or two very small points where the tissues feel most tense and cause the most pain. These may be as small as a pinhead, and the therapist needs to concentrate his attention to find them. The patient can help if he uses a sliding scale of 1–5 for the amount of pain and reports on what he is feeling as the therapist palpates.

Once a point has been found, the pressure should be slowly increased until it is just within the patient's pain tolerance. If increased too quickly, a reflex tightening will occur and the technique will not work. If this starts to happen, the pressure should be eased off so that the tissues can relax, and it can then be increased again more slowly. Increasing the pressure during an exhalation may also help, as the body naturally relaxes more during this part of the breathing cycle.

Everything possible must be done to help the patient deal with the pain. Apart from the digit being used to apply the technique, the other fingers, hand and/or forearm can also be in gentle contact with the patient. Not only will this give the therapist better sensitivity and control, but it also gives the patient more comfort too. It is sometimes possible to use the other hand or arm to apply some body-rocking at the same time to further aid relaxation. Even the tone of the therapist's voice can help, by being calm and supportive while encouraging the patient to relax and breathe deeply into the pain.

The deep pressure is held for up to 90 seconds, and during that time the patient should be asked three or four times if the pain is reducing (even though the therapist may feel and know that it is). When it does, the patient should be encouraged and told that this is good. If the pain starts to increase, the technique should be stopped as this suggests the possibility of some acute inflammation.

The points treated are often the same as acupressure points, and indeed NMT and acupressure are similar in many ways. So the therapist

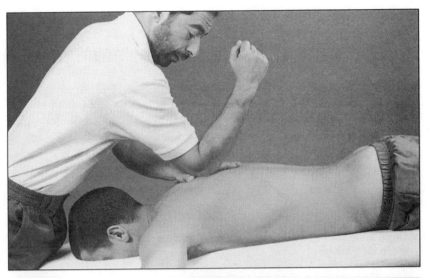

NMT with the elbow into a point in the thoracic spine.

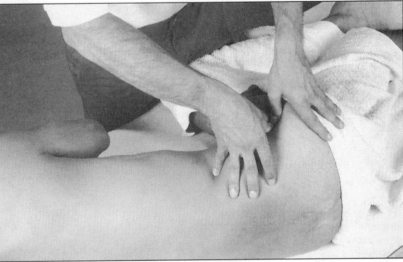

NMT with the thumbs into a point in the tensor fascia lata muscle.

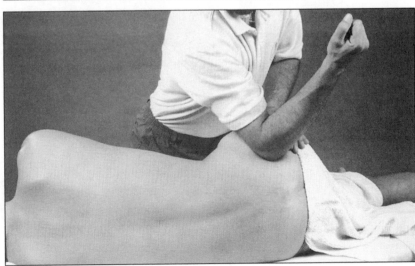

NMT with the elbow into a point near the piriformis origin.

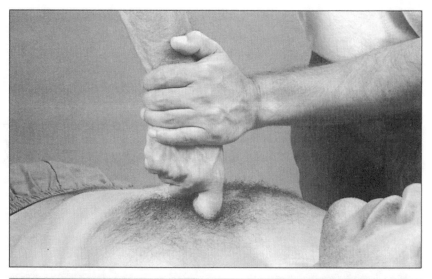

NMT with the knuckle into a point in the intercostal muscle.

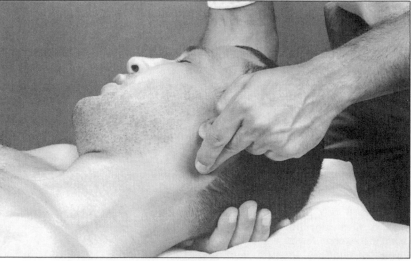

NMT with the fingertip into a point near the sternocleidomastoid attachment.

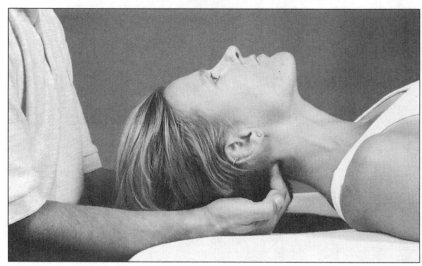

NMT with the fingertips to points in the sub-occipital region.

may actually feel a pulse, or the patient may feel referred sensations elsewhere in the body (see Chapter 15).

NMT need not be applied just in this static way, for friction and stroking movements can also be made. In fact, for the massage therapist it is more a case of adding the NMT principle to deep massage techniques. This combines the release of tension with the breakdown of adhesions and stretching the fibres, and can be extremely powerful. But this must be done very slowly to allow the patient time to anticipate the stroke and keep relaxing into it.

If there is excessive tension in a muscle, it will pull tighter through the tendon and its attachment. Deep palpation will identify the same painful points in these structures, too. What makes treatment near the attachments more significant are the golgi tendon organs (which are located in the tendon close to the attachment). These are load-detectors, which feed information to the central nervous system and help regulate muscle tension. NMT pressure here will inhibit the neural messages from the organ, which can cause relaxation throughout the whole muscle.

This is particularly useful when trying to release tension in very deep muscles, which it may be difficult to reach directly. It is usually possible to work along the bone to find the attachment, and NMT here will have a beneficial reflex effect throughout the muscle. For example, it is possible to relax the deep hip extensor muscles by working along the iliac crest. NMT applied along the lateral border of the sternum can release the intercostal muscles lying beneath the breast tissue. Treating the attachments can even be used to relax a traumatized muscle, which will not tolerate direct physical treatment.

Muscle Energy Technique (MET)

MET is a collective name for a variety of techniques that stretch, strengthen or break down fibrous adhesions. A muscle energy technique is one in which the patient's own effort and movement, rather than that of the therapist, provides the primary force in treating the problem.

Imbalance Nearly all musculoskeletal problems involve an imbalance, with some muscles being weak and others being strong and tight. This may be the primary component of the injury or it may be the secondary result of a joint problem, but in either case it needs to be correctly dealt with. An imbalance is not always the easiest thing to assess, as every individual has his own unique balance of strengths and weaknesses, due to adaptation to his individual lifestyle.

Where there is a clear dysfunction, the tight or weak muscles are usually quite easy to identify by observation, palpation and testing the range of movement. Less dysfunctional and chronic conditions are less easy to assess and as well as looking for physical signs, a degree of experience and intuition may also be necessary. As MET is a very safe technique, therapists sometimes use it to stretch or strengthen particular muscles and then see what functional improvement occurs.

There is some predictability in the muscles that become tight and those that become weak in response to stress or injury:

- Tight: postural, static and aerobic muscles
- Weak: anaerobic, speed and power muscles

Opposing muscles The muscular system works through opposing patterns of activity, and when one muscle (or group) contracts, its opposing muscles automatically relax through *reciprocal inhibition*. Messages are transmitted to inform the central nervous system (CNS) that the muscle is under tension. The reflex response to this is to inhibit the nerve input to the opposing muscle, which causes it to relax. This is an extremely important reflex, which enables the body to move freely and efficiently.

A muscle that is tight can transmit the same message to the CNS as if it were contracting. So tension in a muscle can create a weakening in its opposing muscle. It can also work the other way round, with a muscle that has become weak through injury causing tension to increase in the opposing muscle. To restore balance it is necessary to stretch the tight muscle first, to remove any inhibition and allow the weak muscle to be strengthened.

Stretching techniques These techniques allow a muscle to be stretched beyond its present capability by inducing a temporary state of relaxation or inhibition. They can work extremely well on muscles that are excessively tight, but cannot be used to achieve hyper-flexibility beyond what would be normal to that person.

There are two different methods of MET stretching based on different principles.

Post-isometric relaxation (PIR)
Immediately following a period of isometric contraction, a muscle becomes inhibited and more relaxed (hypotonic) for about 5–10 seconds before its normal tone returns. During this induced period of deep relaxation the tissues can be passively stretched further and held in this new position for 10–15 seconds, to allow the nervous system to accept the new tissue length. The increased elasticity achieved by this will be permanent, providing the original cause of the problem has been resolved and stretching exercises are performed for a few days.

Reciprocal inhibition (RI)
When a muscle contracts, its opposing muscle automatically relaxes. Immediately the contraction is released, and before the opposing muscle has time to return to its normal tone, it can be stretched in the same way as with the PIR method.

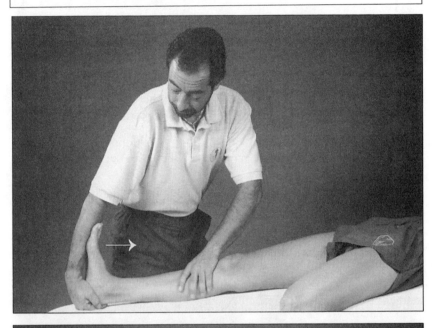

Gastrocnemius: fixing the knee in extension with one hand, the other hand grasps around the heel and, with the forearm, moves the patient's foot into dorsiflexion. The soleus can be done in the same way, but with the knee flexed.

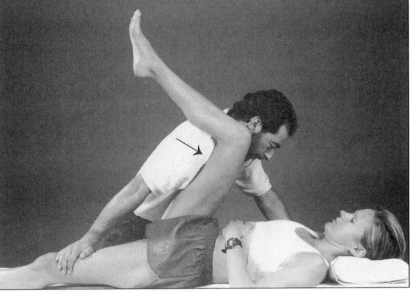

Gluteus maximus: the therapist uses his shoulder to flex the hip, controlling and supporting the movement through his leading (left) arm. The other hand can press down lightly on the patient's other leg to prevent any pelvic movement.

Gluteus medius and minimus: the therapist uses his upper body to lean against the whole length of the patient's thigh, which stops the pelvis lifting off the couch. The limb is stretched diagonally across the patient's body towards the opposite shoulder.

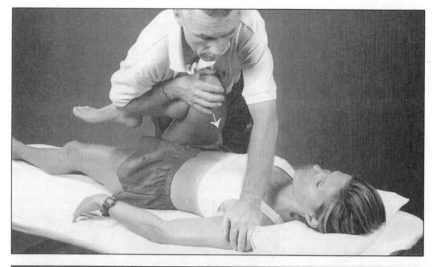

Hamstrings: the therapist applies some pressure with his lower hand to fix the knee in extension, and then raises the leg to stretch the muscle. The therapist can use his knee to keep the other leg down and prevent the pelvis moving.

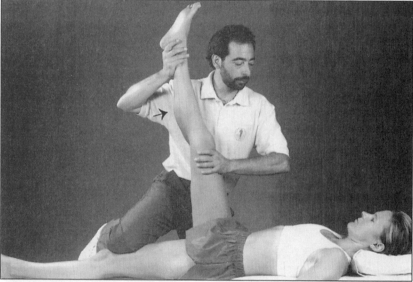

Hip extensor and rotator muscles: the patient's knee can be guided through a variety of flexed and adducted/abducted positions and the therapist can also use his other hand, at the ankle, to add rotation. Rather than affecting a single muscle, this works many muscles involved in a functional pattern. The technique can be applied in whichever direction movement is restricted.

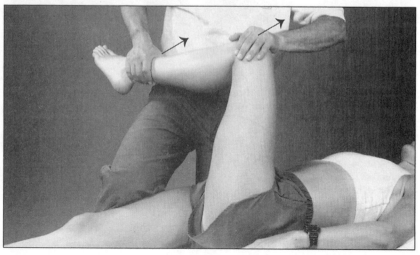

The RI principle can be put to other uses, too. If a muscle is tight, deep massage techniques may be difficult to perform and not very effective. But if the patient is made to contract the opposing muscle at the same time, then the tissues being treated relax and the results are very much better.

Methods of operation   Initially the two stretching MET methods are the same. The therapist passively stretches the tight muscle, by moving the associated joint, until a position is reached that causes the first sign of a mild stretch, but there must be no actual pain. This position is commonly called the *barrier,* and it should be fixed by the therapist so that no movement can occur.

Applying the stretch in exactly the right direction requires some skill. Although there may be a good standard way of stretching a particular large muscle group, the problem area may be only a small part of one muscle within the group. It may, therefore, require subtle changes in position and angle to focus the stretch into exactly the right part.

The accuracy of this holding position at the barrier is crucial to the success of the technique. Usually the therapist would have palpated the area to identify the tension, and the patient will have felt this. So the patient should be asked if he feels the mild stretch in the same place. It is also common for the patient to allow the initial stretch to be taken a little too far, just beyond the barrier. To check that the position is correct, if the patient slightly contracts the stretched muscle the feeling of a mild stretch should disappear; if it increases, the patient has either contracted too quickly, too strongly or his holding position is too stretched.

Many patients seem to have a 'no pain, no gain' attitude to treatment, especially because pain is an integral part of many other massage techniques. It is worth reassuring the patient that it is *good* when the stretch sensation seems to disappear.

The force of contraction used in these techniques need not be great, and they can work on a very subtle level: moderate (less than 50 per cent) isometric contraction for a sustained period (about 10 seconds), resulting in a muscle relaxation afterwards lasting 5–10 seconds. Strong contractions for shorter periods do not normally work as well. It seems that it is time, rather than intensity, that governs the nervous system in this situation. When working with painful neck conditions, for example, having the patient just look in a particular direction creates the slightest isometric contraction in the neck muscles, and even this can be enough to make the technique work. The patient should contract the muscle slowly, building it up gradually over 1–2 seconds. After a steady, sustained contraction it should be released slowly also.

Relaxation is the key to MET and can be enhanced with a breathing technique. The body generally relaxes more when exhaling than when inhaling, so the patient can take a deep breath in and then exhale freely at the same time as the relaxation element of the technique is performed.

It is equally important for the therapist to relax into the technique, as he is also using his body as an integral part of it. He needs to have a good stance and be well supported, and he can use the couch and even sometimes lean on the patient for greater balance. Breathing in time with the patient, and trying to relax as the stretch is applied, can also add an extra dimension.

Method 1 (PIR)

The patient isometrically contracts the muscle that is being stretched, using only moderate force. If a joint has to be *flexed* to achieve the stretch, then the patient should attempt to *extend* it against the fixed resistance.

After holding for 10 seconds, the muscle should be allowed 1–2 seconds to relax fully, then it should slowly and steadily be stretched further until a new barrier position is reached. This position should be held comfortably for 5–10 seconds.

Method 2 (RI)

The patient contracts the opposing muscle to the one being stretched. If the joint is *flexed* to stretch the muscle, the patient should attempt to *flex* even further against resistance.

At the same time the patient releases the contraction, the muscle is simultaneously stretched and then held at the new barrier position.

These techniques can be repeated many times on an individual muscle, until no further progress is being made (usually about three times). On the final application the new position should be held for about 20 seconds.

Deciding whether to use the PIR or the RI method can be very simple. When the barrier position is fixed, the patient is asked to try the technique in both directions. If one feels uncomfortable, then only the other should be used. If neither causes any discomfort, then the two methods can be used alternately.

Apart from this, there are particular situations where one method or the other should *not* be used:

• PIR (Method 1) should not be used on a muscle that has recently sustained an acute injury. The tissues could be re-torn if held in a stretched position and the patient tries to contract. But the RI method works extremely well in these situations.
• RI (Method 2) should not be used if, when the muscle is stretched to the barrier position, the opposing muscle is put into a very shortened position. Any attempt to contract this opposing muscle could cause it to go into spasm (cramp), as it will be unable to contract in this shortened state.

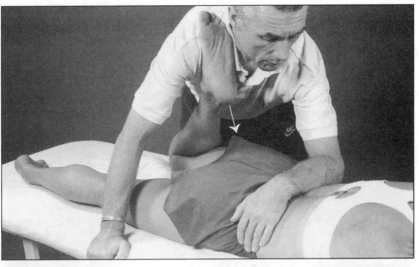

Quadriceps: with one arm across the back of the hips to prevent movement, the therapist can use his shoulder to flex the knee.

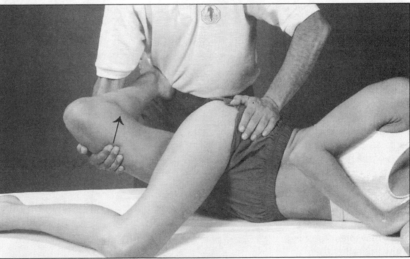

Tensor fascia lata: in a side-lying position, the patient's lower leg can be elevated to stretch the muscle.

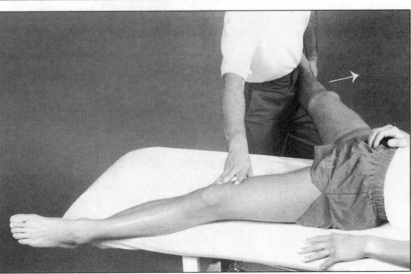

Adductors: preventing movement in one leg, the other can be abducted to stretch the muscle. The degree of rotation in the leg can be altered to work different parts of the group.

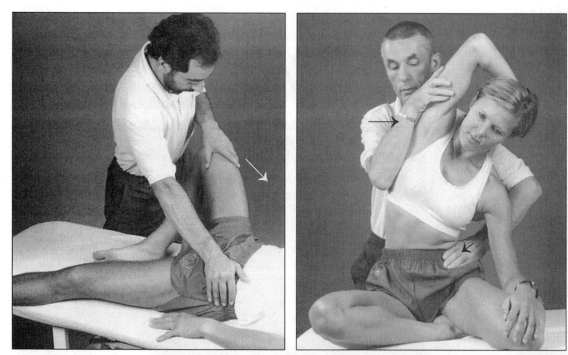

Above (left): Adductors: with varying degrees of hip and knee flex, the therapist can abduct the leg to stretch different parts of the muscle group.

Above (right): Quadratus lumborum: the therapist is using his lower hand on the iliac crest to prevent pelvic movement (pushing it inwards rather than down). The other hand is used to guide the patient into a side-bent position to stretch the muscle.

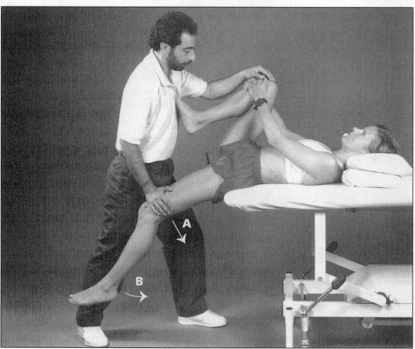

A) Iliopsoas muscles: with the patient lying supine with his buttock just off the end of the couch, the therapist presses down on the knee. Both patient and therapist must ensure that the hip of the other leg is kept flexed at all times to protect the lower back (slight neck flexion also helps this).

B) Rectus femoris: keeping the knee fixed, with a mild stretch on the hip, the therapist can use his shin or foot to press against the patient's lower leg to stretch the muscle.

The stretching techniques described here are based on the conventional clinical situation on a treatment couch. But MET has great potential when applied off the couch using functional movements. If a patient says it hurts or feels stiff when making a particular movement, such as turning in a chair or looking over a shoulder, get them to perform this movement and stop when they start to feel discomfort (the barrier). The therapist should hold him firmly in this position and the patient should then attempt to move further in one direction and/or back in the other direction. Rather than working with individual muscles, this functional approach works with whole patterns of muscular activity, which can have far more significant results.

The PIR method of stretching tight muscles can easily be adapted for self-use, by performing a mild stretch and then contracting gently against it. Many sportsmen now use it regularly as part of their stretching technique.

Strengthening (toning) technique

Muscles may become weak because of a combination of injury, lack of use and nerve inhibition. Once any root cause of the problem has been resolved, then normal use, or exercise, should be able to restore its strength. However, the body learns to adapt and compensate for small areas of weakness. Thanks to the complexity of the muscular system, we can alter movement patterns so that we avoid using weak muscles but can still perform our daily activities. So the weak muscle does not get the exercise it needs and does not improve. There may, of course, be other consequences to these altered patterns elsewhere in the body, too.

Whether it is the cause or the consequence, the nerve stimulation to a weak muscle reduces and after a time conductivity through the nerve becomes poor. It takes time and effort actually to strengthen muscle fibre, but nerve conductivity improves very quickly when stimulated. This is why there is initially great improvement in apparent strength when starting a new sport or activity – it is the increased nerve stimulation, rather than true strength, that causes this.

By isolating the specific muscle that is weak and making it work (contract), the nerves are stimulated and this rapidly improves its function. In fact, a real improvement can usually be felt after only four or five contractions, and the functional effect can sometimes be quite remarkable. The patient immediately feels that there is better movement and therefore uses it more normally. With better (normal) use, the strengthening effects can continue and can lead to full function and balance.

Sometimes a patient will have a severe and progressively weakening situation, as lack of use and weakness both act on each other. A single treatment can sometimes completely reverse this into a progressively strengthening situation.

Method of application

The muscle should be stretched slightly, but not as far as the barrier to start with. The therapist applies a controlled force and the patient

Levator scapula and posterior neck muscles: with one hand fixing the shoulder down, the other hand supports firmly around the back of the head and moves the neck though a variety of flexed and rotated positions. The technique can be applied in whichever direction movement is restricted. (Greater support and control are achieved if the patient's head is resting against the therapist's abdomen.)

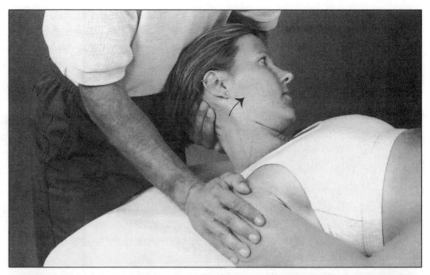

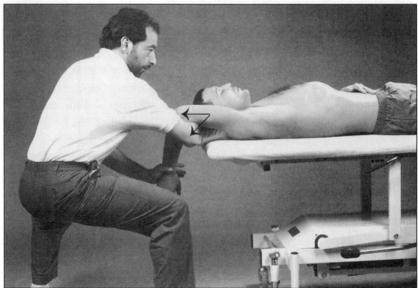

Serratus anterior and arm adductors: linking the inner elbows together, the therapist can pull back to stretch the muscles.

pushes or pulls against it. This must be done through a carefully determined range of movement to ensure that exactly the right muscle is used. The patient should first use concentric contractions, which are safer, and then, as tone improves, eccentric contractions can be introduced as well.

It is important to concentrate first on the quality of movement by developing the fullest range, rather than the greatest force. So the technique should start slowly with light pressure and not build up so quickly that the range begins to reduce.

In long-term, chronic situations nerve conductivity may have become so poor that the patient has real difficulty in creating any movement and feels that he does not even know *how* to move it. The therapist should then start with passive movements, with the patient seeing,

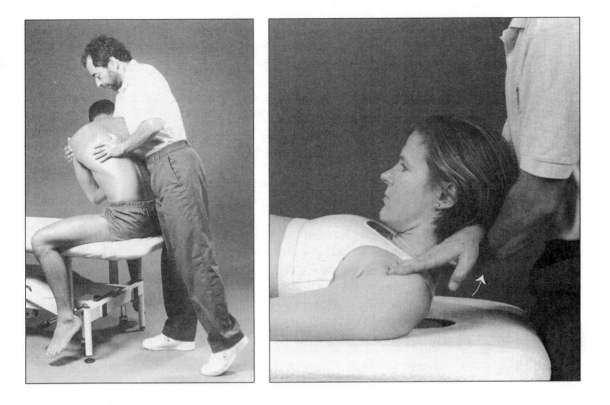

Above (left): Back muscles: with the patient sitting, the therapist can guide him into a variety of flexed and rotated positions. The technique can be applied in whichever direction movement is restricted.

Above (right): Posterior neck muscles: with the hands gently pressing the shoulders down, the therapist can use his forearms to flex the neck.

feeling and experiencing the movement first. He may then be able to assist this movement, before progressing to the full active method.

When weakness affects small muscles that control joint movement, especially around the ankle, several muscles are usually involved to varying degrees, so the joint needs to be worked in all possible directions. To improve stability (proprioception) of the joint, the therapist should constantly change the direction in which he wants the patient to push or pull. After a short time the patient should close his eyes and just move in response to the feel of the therapist's hand.

Where a joint injury has occurred the associated muscles will rapidly lose strength. In the initial acute stage of treatment, this strengthening technique can be used in a slightly different way. The therapist can fix the joint statically in a comfortable position, so that damaged tissues are not disturbed, and get the patient to contract the muscles by attempting to move in all directions. When movement becomes possible, the full active technique can be used very effectively as an integral part of rehabilitation.

MET to break adhesions and fibrosis

Muscle tissue may become fibrotic through tension and the formation of adhesions through micro-trauma. The fibres become matted together, and as they cannot glide independently the area will not function (contract or be stretched). To break these bonds a very powerful force needs to be created between the fibres to pull them apart. The strongest way of doing this is to get the fibres themselves to attempt a contraction (shortening), while at the same time the muscle as a whole is being stretched (lengthened).

This can be achieved with a forced eccentric contraction. Here the patient forcefully contracts the muscle, from a shortened position, and the therapist applies a greater force to overcome this and stretches the muscle out at the same time. So if the patient contracts a muscle that extends a joint, the therapist should force it into flexion. This produces a very strong shearing force between the fibres, which breaks the adhesive bonds and enables them to function normally again.

This MET technique is rather drastic and can cause considerable pain. Care must be taken not to use too much force, as this could actually tear fibres. It is not used very often, because other massage techniques usually deal with fibrosis well enough, but in extremely chronic situations it can produce excellent results.

Proprioceptive neuromuscular facilitation (PNF)

(Proprioceptive: receiving nerve stimulation; neuromuscular: relating to nerves and muscles; facilitation: promoting a natural process.)

This is in fact an advanced form of MET. It uses the same methods to change the muscle tone, but works through complete movement patterns, which achieve a wider and more integrated re-balancing. The MET described here deals only with local situations, although with experience the therapist may naturally begin to develop this broader understanding.

Soft Tissue Release (STR)

This is a new technique that is becoming popular among sports massage therapists in the UK. It can produce a quick and effective result in releasing local areas of severe soft tissue tension, hence the name STR. It is not a pure technique based on its own theory, but rather a hybrid that combines several techniques.

Friction

With a conventional friction technique the tissues remain still and passive and the movement is made by the therapist. But with STR the therapist applies passive pressure and the movement is made functionally (active or passive). The friction breaks the adhesions binding the fibres, and the movement causes this to happen in exactly the right direction that is needed to re-align them so that they can provide proper function.

Stretch

With standard stretching methods it is possible that due to the elasticity of the muscle as a whole, the stretch may not effectively reach a specific area of tension within it. The majority of the muscle fibres will be healthy and elastic and may be able to accommodate full extension of the muscle without causing the tense area to be stretched. That is why tension can develop even with a good stretching programme, the hamstrings being a prime example. Similarly, the range of movement structurally possible at a joint may prevent it moving far enough to stretch areas of tension within the muscle; for example the biceps brachii cannot stretch fully, due to the limited range of the elbow extension.

With STR, a local area of tight and adhered fibres is locked still by an applied pressure, and the tissues are stretched away from that point. This focuses the stretch to just those tissues and is extremely effective and produces immediate results. The tissues on the other side of the locked-in pressure (away from the stretched side) do not get disturbed at all, which makes it safe and possible to release muscle tension very close to an acute area of damage.

Neuromuscular The points where the pressure is applied are often the same as those used in an NMT situation. Although it is only held for a few seconds in STR, this still has a good neuromuscular effect. The patient still has to relax into the pain but also has to overcome the instinct to contract the muscle by allowing it to lengthen instead. It also helps the nervous system relax the tissues through a range of movement, rather than in just one position.

Diagnostic With the normal palpatory method, the tissues remain still and passive and the fingers glide through them to assess any textural changes. But with STR the pressure is static and the tissues themselves are moved. Although this may not seem very significant, it does help to be able to feel an area in these two different ways. Where there may be several muscle layers going in different directions, feeling the movement of the tissues helps determine which level (or muscle) may be involved.

The technique STR is most commonly used on muscles but can also be highly effective on tendons and ligaments. Working on small areas, a strongly supported thumb is normally used, but on larger areas the fist or heel of the palm usually works better.

The basic method is to start with the muscle relaxed and held in a shortened position by moving the associated joint. Deep focused pressure should be applied directly into the adhered fibres to fix them in position. The muscle is then stretched (passively) away from this fixed point by moving the joint.

A common mistake is to allow the pressure point to move with the tissues as they are stretched, but this takes away all the effect. The pressure needs to applied with sufficient force to resist and prevent the local tissues from moving. As the stretch takes place, the pressure point can be drawn a couple of inches (or a few centimetres) in the opposite direction without reducing the pressure, which achieves an even greater local stretch.

An easy way to think of the technique is:

- The lock: the area of adhered fibres
- The key: deep focused pressure (into the lock)
- Open the door: stretch the tissues away. $\longrightarrow$

A big muscle that feels generally tight can be treated first with large pressure points, using the hand or fist working up and down the muscle to release superficial tension. Then deeper pressure can be focused through the thumb, working systematically through the area. The technique is repeated many times in succession as the area is covered, and it helps relaxation if this follows a smooth rhythm.

This method can be enhanced by using active and resisted movements, instead of passive ones, to stretch the muscle. To do this the patient must contract the antagonist that reciprocally inhibits (relaxes) the muscle being treated. So instead of the therapist moving the joint, he applies a resistance and has the patient force the movement. The tissues can also be stretched away from the pressure point using deep massage strokes made with the other hand. This is useful when it is not convenient to move the joint, for example when treating the gluteal muscles in the prone lying position where hip flexion to stretch the muscle would be impossible.

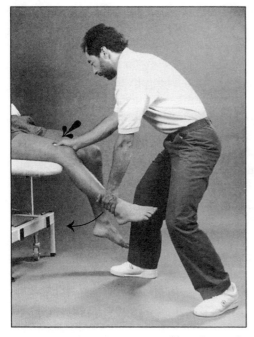

Quadriceps: pressure applied with the thumb into the muscle as it is stretched by flexing the knee.

This describes the basic application of the STR technique, but these principles (lock, key and door) can be put to use in a wide variety of ways. Although STR is very good in the conventional treatment situation on a therapy couch, its real versatility is seen off the couch. It can be used sitting, standing or in any position and, being just as simple through clothes, can be done anywhere.

Wherever there is a lock in the tissues, insert the key and open the door. Here are some examples:

- In the rhomboid area: with the therapist facing the back of the seated patient, he should press firmly into a tender point. The patient should then reach forward with his arm as far as possible to draw the scapula forward and stretch the tissues away from the point. This can be repeated several times, using different points and with the patient stretching his arm forward in different directions.
- In the upper trapezius: with the key in the lock, the patient can move his head and neck, and/or pull his elbow down. This can stretch the tissues on either or both sides of the point.

STR can also be used in self-treatment. For the hamstrings, sit on a table with the hands under the thigh. The fingers can be pressed up into the point and a leg extension will stretch the tissues away from it.

Hamstrings: pressure applied with the ulnar border of the hand into the muscle as it is stretched by extending the knee.

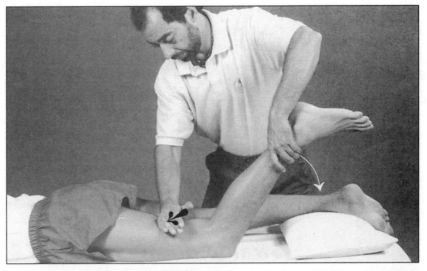

Pectoralis major: pressure applied with the fingers into the muscle as it is stretched by lowering the arm.

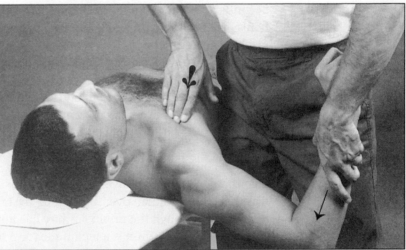

Adductors: pressure applied with the fingers into the muscle as the leg is abducted, with varying degrees of flexion and rotation.

The most simple way to use STR is as follows: if a patient says it hurts *here* (lock) when I do *this* movement (door), the therapist has only to put the key into the lock. This technique is very useful with sportsmen, who can reproduce the action concerned while the pressure is applied.

STR is an innovative technique that challenges the flair and ingenuity of the therapist but, like all other techniques, it requires much practice to develop the handling skills necessary for success. It may not be able to deal with the root cause of many chronic conditions, but its effect on muscle tension and scar tissue from soft tissue injury is excellent and gives immediate results. For this reason it is becoming a very popular pre-event technique in sports situations.

Strain-Counterstrain (SCS)

Secondary tension builds up very quickly around damaged muscle fibres, even on a microscopic level. This is part of the natural defence mechanism of the body, which acts to protect the injury from further damage and to stop it spreading. This can also occur through a protective spasm, where a large area of muscle contracts to prevent a movement that would be likely to cause injury. The secondary tension restricts movement and any attempt to stretch this out is likely to re-inforce the protective reflex and cause greater contraction and pain.

This tension restricts local blood-flow so it does not help the healing process. It can also adversely affect normal movement patterns and may become habitual over time, and dysfunctional symptoms may remain even though the original injury has long since recovered.

Strain-Counterstrain is a technique (developed by Lawrence Jones, DO, in America) that can simply and painlessly release this tension:

- As already stated, the tension and pain will increase if stretching is attempted. So instead the muscle is shortened by passively moving further in the direction of the contraction, until a position of greatest ease and comfort is found.
- Held in this comfortably relaxed position for about 90 seconds, there is a calming effect on the neurological reporting stations in the muscle spindles, which control tension, and this can switch off the protective spasm.
- The muscle can then be passively stretched beyond its previously restricted range. This movement, however, must be done very slowly and passively, as any active assistance by the patient is likely to cause the spasm to return.
- Once the length has been restored, it should be held in this new position for up to 60 seconds to allow the tissues and the nervous system to adapt to the situation.

This method can be extremely effective with gross movement problems, such as a stiff neck caused by whiplash, or muscle spasm in the back. For example, if a patient is locked in a side-bent position and unable to straighten up due to spasm, he should be held (or placed) in a *more* bent position in which he can completely relax. After about 90 seconds, when the spasm has released, the patient should be slowly and passively moved into a straightened position and allowed to rest there for up to a minute. If the spasm is the only thing causing the restriction and there is no other underlying damage, this technique can sometimes appear to have almost miraculous results.

SCS can also be used on smaller areas of secondary tension, which do not cause such gross movement problems. With the muscle resting in a lengthened position, the tissues should be palpated to find an acutely tender point within it. These will usually be the same as NMT points. A moderate, constant pressure should be applied into this point to cause mild discomfort, which the patient uses as a monitor for the technique. The muscle is then slowly and passively shortened by the therapist, and the patient reports any changes in discomfort felt at the pressure point. The therapist should stop at the position where the patient feels the *greatest ease*. This position is held for a period and then passively and slowly lengthened in the same way as already described.

When dealing with a problem in, say, the hamstrings, this technique is relatively simple. With the patient's leg lying extended on the couch (prone), the therapist presses into the tender point in the muscle until the patient reports that he feels mild discomfort. The therapist then uses his other hand to raise the ankle slowly, to flex the knee, and so shorten the muscle. When the position of greatest ease is felt at the pressure point, the therapist fixes and holds this position. The muscle must be returned to its resting length very slowly to enable the patient to stay relaxed.

In more complex muscle areas, like the hip, there may be several muscles in spasm and it may be difficult to determine the particular range of movement to work through. In this situation the patient should be placed in a position that allows the greatest variety of movement so that they can all be tried. With the hip muscles, a side-lying position works very well. While applying pressure into a tender point in the muscles, the joint should be moved through flexion and extension, stopping at the point of greatest ease. From this position it can then be moved through adduction and abduction, stopping at the point of ease, and then rotation and circumduction can be added. Sometimes the therapist may find himself in an uncomfortable position when reaching the final counterstrain position, and he should then move into a comfortable position first so that he can hold the technique for the 90 seconds required. For the shoulder muscles it is often better to sit the patient in a chair so that all ranges of movement can be worked through.

This technique is highly effective in relieving local spasm, especially around an injury. But in the post-acute or chronic stage, or if other factors causing the spasm remain unresolved, the effects of the technique may not last very long. However, in terms of treatment, this temporary release of tension may enable the therapist to get deeper into the area and achieve better results on the whole problem.

Although the SCS technique itself is very simple, good results are not easy to achieve. The patient's complete relaxation is needed throughout the operation, and everything must be done to try and achieve this. Good quality of handling by the therapist is vital, and even the right tone of voice can help. Patients who are used to deep massage may expect good results only with techniques that cause pain, and it is important to assure them that this technique works, because there is no pain. Before making any movement it is also helpful to tell the patient what is happening and to stay completely relaxed, so that there is no element of surprise.

Connective Tissue Manipulation (CTM)

Treatment aimed specifically at the connective tissue began in Germany in the 1930s and was developed for the treatment of medical disorders. It was realized then that a peripheral nerve that supplies an organ also supplies a particular segment of the skin and subcutaneous layers. The plasticity, and other properties, of these tissues were found to be poor when there was dysfunction in the associated organ. Treating the connective tissue in this segment appeared to affect the autonomic nerve supply (sympathetic and parasympathetic) along the peripheral network and to improve the condition of the organ. Traditional Connective Tissue Manipulation (CTM) books have clear charts showing the areas of skin that relate to the specific organs, and the pattern and direction of strokes used to treat their dysfunction.

Connective tissue is also believed to be important in psycho/emotional therapy situations. As a continual membrane, the surface tissues directly connect all the way through to the brain. An emotional state can affect the condition of the connective tissue in the brain and, over time, spread to other areas and lead to physical symptoms there.

Myo facial techniques

In the treatment of musculoskeletal problems, the connective tissue of primary concern is the myo (muscle) fascia. This binds the muscle fibres into bundles and compartments, and binds all these together to form the whole muscle. The outer layer of fascia makes up the muscle sheath, which maintains the overall shape and is smooth on the outside so that the muscle can move freely and independently of other structures. It is not contractile tissue but does have – or should have – the same elasticity as the muscle.

The quality of the connective tissue can generally be assessed by the plasticity of the skin and subcutaneous layers. Thickened, adhered fascia is less mobile, and the skin will glide only a short distance before feeling tight. With healthy tissue it is amazing how far it can comfortably be stretched in all directions.

The fascia is subject to trauma through over-stretching or impact (it does not get strained, as it is not contractile), and scar tissue and adhesions can form in the same way as with muscle tissue. The main problem, however, comes from chronic changes as a result of long-term stress (physical, postural or emotional). The fascia thickens and becomes more fibrous, which makes it less mobile and reduces its permeability. This affects the function of the underlying muscle and may restrict its free movement. And, if the interstitial fluid cannot pass freely through the fascia, the muscle may not get an adequate supply of oxygen and nutrients and will be less able to eliminate metabolic waste material.

As well as releasing excessive tension or thickening in the fascia, CTM techniques affect the autonomic nervous system through a neurofascial reflex. This stimulates local blood-flow, which can clearly be seen after treatment, as the skin should appear very red.

Methods of operation CTM is normally applied through the tips and pads of the fingers, which must be strongly supported. A good grip with the skin is essential, so there must be no oil present. The technique is even sometimes performed through a towel, to provide stronger contact without the need for too much pressure.

The initial movement is simply pressure into the skin and subcutaneous layer, which stops at the level of the muscle. This requires good tactile skill and needs much practice to be able to feel the subtle difference in tissue density and know exactly how deep to press. At this level, any stroke will move the tissues over the fascia, providing the skin does not slide under the finger. If the fascia is in good condition, the skin will slide smoothly, but if it is thick and fibrous it will not.

With this pressure constantly maintained, a stroke is applied at a slow, steady speed to take up the available 'slack' in the skin and subcutaneous layer. The skin should not be allowed to slide under the fingers at all, and the only sensation the patient should experience during this initial part of the stroke is that of touch. When resistance is felt in the pliability of the tissues, without increasing the depth of pressure, the stroke should be forced on for an inch or so (a few more centimetres). This should create a mild scratching or burning sensation felt by the patient on a level deeper than the skin. This is because friction is being created between the fascia and the subcutaneous layer, as they are drawn across each other. This releases tension and breaks adhesions affecting the fascia. At the end of the stroke the pressure should be released so that the skin returns to its normal position before starting the next stroke.

Longer strokes can also be applied using a very small amount of oil to allow the skin to slide slightly under the fingers. After the shorter

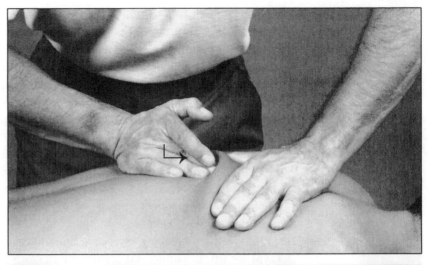

The fingers move the skin and subcutaneous layers over the muscle fascia.

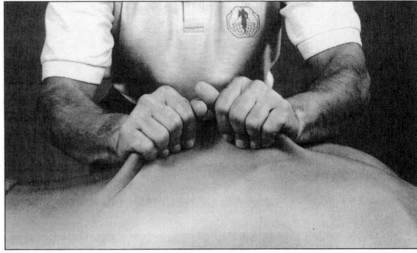

The hands can be used to grasp and lift the skin and subcutaneous layers away from the underlying muscle.

stroke has been forced on, maintaining the same traction, the therapist should continue along, with the skin slowly passing under his fingers. The same deep scratching sensation should be felt by the patient throughout this extended stroke.

Applications   This technique may be used at the start of a treatment if the tissues are very tense and feel congested, with poor skin plasticity. In this situation regular massage techniques may be difficult to perform, as it is hard to pick up the tissues and may also feel quite uncomfortable to the patient. Working first on the connective tissue in this way can be very relaxing, can stimulate blood-flow and release congestion, making normal massage easier to perform afterwards. Any part of the body may require this attention, but the most common area to benefit is the back.

When CTM is applied slowly it can be extremely relaxing, but when done vigorously it is highly stimulating. This can be very useful at the end of a treatment to 'wake' the patient up.

When treating the back, as well as the standard finger method, the heel or whole palm of the hand can be used (through a towel for grip) to move the skin over the muscle in all directions. Another method is to grasp a handful of skin between the fingers and the heel of the palm so that the hand is making a half-fist. The mass of skin that has been picked up can then be drawn back and forth across the muscle quite forcefully.

The muscles on the lateral side of the leg (tensor fascia lata, iliotibial band, vastas lateralis, tibialis anterior and peroneal muscles) naturally have a fairly thick fascia, which responds well to CTM, which should be considered as a regular massage technique here. This can be effectively done with the heel of the palm and using a towel for better grip. The skin layer is thin here, so it does not require much pressure to reach the fascial layer, and the difficulty is to stay at this level and not increase the pressure into the leg during the stroke. One or two strokes should be made up the leg to feel how far the skin will go before the fascia binds. Having tested this 'end-stop', a third stroke should be applied very vigorously to force the tissues beyond that point. This technique does cause a sharp, sudden pain (be warned), but this itself may have a strong neurofascial effect.

One other important area for CTM treatment is the chest. Chronic tension (usually postural) is common here and the fascia plays a major part in this. Very deep, long CTM stokes along the intercostal muscles, above the belly of the pectorals and below the breast are highly effective and can lead to quite profound changes in posture and breathing. But they must be done slowly due to the pain involved. In this particular situation, CTM and the NMT technique for the chest area are virtually the same.

Other variations To release the deep fascia between muscle and bone, the limb should be positioned so that the muscle is relaxed and shortened. The whole muscle should be grasped firmly and pushed or pulled transversely away from the bone. The tissues should be held in the stretched position for a few moments to have real benefit. With chronic tension, a gentle thrust can also be applied to break any adhesions.

To mobilize the fascia between muscles and other soft tissues, fairly deep pressure is applied into the tissues between the muscles (or its compartments), ligaments or tendons. This is held for a few seconds to allow the tissues to relax. The patient then moves the tissues by contracting or relaxing the muscle. As this is done, the therapist applies the CTM stroke across the fascia. As well as releasing tension, this movement helps the collagen fibres of the fascia to re-align better.

As CTM can also be done through clothing it has much potential when working outdoors or at sports events.

15 Acupressure

Alastair N. Greetham, MCSP

Introduction

Acupressure therapy, sometimes called needle-finger therapy, uses manual pressure to stimulate points on the body, instead of the insertion of needles. The advantages are obvious: acupressure is safe, can be performed almost anywhere and requires no special equipment save the practitioner's hands, knowledge and skills.

It is beyond the scope of this chapter to look at the topic in great detail. It is hoped, however, that a consideration of some of the main concepts will give an insight into another way of perceiving the body and the issue of health.

Most people are familiar with the simplest therapeutic use of pressure. When pain is felt, an immediate and reflexive action is to rub, press or hold the injured area until the pain subsides. In trigger-point therapy, pressing on tender points around an area of the body helps to release pain and tension in the tissues. These localized tender places are referred to in Chinese medicine as Ashi points and are important in the treatment of musculoskeletal disorders.

Stimulating local points is the most basic use of acupressure and probably the most easily accessible for those accustomed to Western methods of treatment. This is, however, only a small part of an ancient system of medical practice that includes needling, herbal therapy, manipulation, exercise, massage and meditation. The vast body of knowledge associated with these practices has, in this century, been somewhat formalized and organized to enable it to be taught outside China. Called Traditional Chinese Medicine (TCM), it is based on its own, internally consistent set of beliefs and philosophies. The principles of treatment are based on an understanding of this way of looking at the world and how it relates to the practice of medicine.

Traditional Chinese Medicine (TCM)

Yin and Yang TCM does not regard the body as a series of independent, mechanical systems. It gives us a picture of a balance of energies, which are interrelated and interdependent. Disease arises from imbalances in the relationships between these forces, or when external factors invade the body. In diagnosis, the practitioner does not seek to identify an ailing organ, a damaged tissue, or even a direct causal factor. His aim is to recognize a pattern of disharmony in the internal environment and, through treatment, to restore balance.

One of the tools that helps to make sense of the complex inter-relationships in the body is the concept of Yin and Yang. The Chinese characters of these words represent respectively the shady and the sunny slopes of a mountain. This philosophical construct represents the duality of interdependent opposition, and the constant movement and change that lie within all natural processes. It lies at the heart of Chinese philosophy and is a wonderfully elegant, theoretical tool for observing and analysing phenomena.

All things can be described in terms of Yin and Yang. The qualities of Yin are said to relate to Water, for example, heaviness, stillness and coldness. Those of Yang relate to Fire, like heat, activity and expansion (Fig. 5). These qualities are opposites but at the same time interdependent and complementary, and they can only be truly defined relative to each other. Heat can only be felt if there is cold, and youth perceived only if there is old age for comparison. These situations are infinitely changeable: a youth is old compared to a new-born baby, and someone with cold hands feels warm to a person who has just come indoors on a freezing day.

Fig. 5: Table showing Yin/Yang qualities

YIN	YANG
Cold	Hot
Night	Day
Darkness	Brightness
Softness	Hardness
Yielding	Resisting
Stillness	Movement
Slow	Quick
Internal	External
Downward	Upward
Passivity	Aggression
Quiet	Loud
Substantial	Ethereal

Einstein's famous equation $E=MC^2$ tells us that energy and what we regard as matter are manifestations of the same phenomena. Yin represents the more substantial, fundamental aspects, while Yang describes the more energetic and active aspects. All things can be described in terms of their Yin and Yang qualities. If we consider ice, water and steam, we see that ice is the most Yin and steam the most Yang. Water is Yang relative to ice but is Yin relative to steam. In between these states exists an infinite number of relative conditions. The Yin/Yang concept does not refer to absolutes; rather it allows us to describe anything in terms of its condition and its relationship to anything else. The description deals with its state at a particular time and relative to its circumstances. Situations are constantly changing, and thus the relative states alter constantly in dynamic systems. This movement is shown in the Yin/Yang symbol (Fig. 6), which portrays the two opposite forces intertwined and transforming into the other in a constant cycle. The small dots show that within Yin there is some Yang, and that within Yang there is some Yin – nothing is absolute.

The Yin/Yang concept is a way to recognize and define patterns within highly complex, dynamic systems. It is a tool for perceiving order within supposed chaos and for allowing recognition of patterns of imbalance.

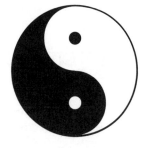

Fig. 6: Yin/Yang symbol

The body is described in terms of Yin and Yang: for example, back (Yang) and front (Yin), upper (Yang) and lower (Ying), external (Yang) and internal (Ying). Each part of the body can be further subdivided into Yin and Yang parts. The internal organs, which in TCM do not just refer to the physiological structures recognized by Western anatomists, are ascribed Yin/Yang characteristics according to their nature and function. Yin and Yang manifest in all aspects of the body, interior and exterior interdependently related, allowing internal imbalances to be treated by working externally on the body. All things exist within this type of relationship; nothing exists in isolation. Man cannot be seen as being separate from his surroundings, but as a part of it and in relationship with it, and therefore influenced by it. Health is seen to be a state where Yin and Yang are in harmony with each other, and the individual exists in sympathy with his environment. Disease occurs when imbalances arise through factors such as poor nutrition, lack or excess of exercise, emotional disturbances or inappropriate lifestyles. Recognition of patterns of disharmony using Yin and Yang is a cornerstone of TCM, and an understanding of the basic tenets will aid further study.

If a person is overweight and his body soft and skin colour pale, then his metabolism may be slow and his circulation poor. The voice may be quiet when he speaks and he may move slowly and tend to complain of the cold. This is a situation where Yin has consumed Yang and thus predominates. The individual's circulation may be sluggish and his system lack a dynamic quality, which may lead to disorders of a deficiency nature, such as poor digestion or a predisposition to infection. A Yang individual may have a hard body and exhibit patterns of muscular tension, may be aggressive and loud when speaking, have a reddish complexion and show an excess of dynamic activity in relation to both movement and bodily function.

When Yin or Yang becomes deficient, we may see a relative excess of the opposite quality in an otherwise healthy individual. A Yang deficiency can give rise to a 'weak cold syndrome', where signs such as poor appetite, fear of cold and a predisposition to catching whatever bug is going round may be apparent. A Yin deficiency can produce a 'weak heat syndrome'. The face may appear reddened, signs of anxiety and agitation may be noted, the individual may complain of difficulty in sleeping and night-sweating (night is a Yin time, and signs such as these show a weakness of Yin and inability to control Yang). It is important to recognize these different scenarios, as it can be seen that they will require different treatments. They are sometimes differentiated by the terms Fullness and Emptiness, or Deficiency and Excess. If we apply this method of thinking to a musculoskeletal situation, an example might be that a muscle is over-used and thus becomes stronger than its opposite (Yang excess). Conversely, it could be that a muscle becomes inhibited or weakened, leading to a relative dominance of its opposite number (Yin deficiency, relative Yang excess). It is crucial to recognize the difference so that appropriate and effective treatment can be administered.

Qi and blood Pronounced 'chee', Qi can be simply described as 'that which does'. It is often referred to in translation as energy, which means vitality and activity, and the capacity to do work. It is not nebulous or fantastic but an absolute reality, and is the manifestation of Yin and Yang in the body. Qi nourishes and warms the body and governs the constant cycles of transformation and transportation that sustain life. It protects the body, warding off pernicious influences. It is the source of all movement and activity, and manifests in the cycles of birth, growth and development. Thus Qi is the energy of change and movement that creates life.

Qi is derived from two sources: Congenital Qi, inherited from our parents, which could be regarded as our life essence, and Acquired Qi. Congenital Qi is finite and when exhausted is gone, and it is seen in all aspects of the body. It is nourished and supported by the renewable resources, the Qi derived from the air we breathe and the food we eat. These combine to form the Meridian Qi, which circulates throughout the body in the channels; the Defensive Qi, which pervades the body, protecting and warming it; and the Nourishing Qi, which moistens and nourishes the body.

A healthy balance of Congenital Qi with abundant Acquired Qi, circulating freely in the channels and organs and throughout all the tissues, ensures health and balance and promotes resistance to disease and injury. Qi is closely linked with blood and could be regarded as its Yang aspect, being responsible for its formation and circulation. Blood provides the nutrition and moistening function that allows Qi to exist. Qi in turn circulates the blood and governs the processes of transformation between the blood and the body, thereby showing the harmonious relationship between the two. It is the Qi and blood that are affected in treatment when the acupressure points are stimulated.

The internal organs The organs of TCM, called the Zang Fu, are defined as much by their functions regarding the vital substances as by their anatomical structure.

There are five Zang (Yin) organs. They control the manufacture and storage of the Qi and blood. Their names are the same as the organs recognized by Western anatomy, but they have much broader functions (Fig. 7). They are each paired with a Fu (Yang) organ, with which an internal channel connects. The Fu organs are generally concerned with receiving food, its containment, digestion and excretion (Fig. 7). The Yin organs are seen to be more fundamental – their activities balanced by the influences of the Yang organs.

The actions of the Zang Fu are distributed in the body via the meridians. These connect to each other at the extremities of the limbs, where the Zang and Fu organs are linked, again creating a circuit for the flow of Qi.

Fig. 7: Paired Yin/Yang organs

ZANG ORGANS (Yin)	FU ORGANS (Yang)
Lung	Large intestine
Spleen	Stomach
Heart	Small intestine
Kidney	Bladder
Liver	Gall bladder

There is another pair of organs, the Heart Constrictor (Yin) and the Triple Heater (Yang). The Heart Constrictor shares the functions of the heart. It completes the picture when we consider the meridian system, as there are six Yin Channels but only five major Yin organs. The Triple Heater is a functional concept linking the actions of the Zang organs at three levels in the body, and is concerned with fluid metabolism. It also completes the picture in terms of the complementary number of Yang channels.

Functions of the Zang organs:

Lung
- Rules Qi and respiration
- Fluid balance and movement
- Protects the exterior (Defensive Qi in the skin and muscles)

Spleen
- Controls all processes of movement and transformation, especially digestion
- Controls blood
- Maintains the quality of the muscles

Heart
- Rules the circulation
- In TCM it is the seat of Mind

Kidney
- Contains the Essence (Inherited Qi)
- Rules the marrow and bones
- Rules the Water

Liver
- Controls the harmonious and free-flowing movement of Qi. This is related especially to:
  a) The emotions
  b) Digestion
  c) Bile
  d) Menstruation
- Stores and regulates blood
- Rules the contractile aspects of muscles

If the organs are healthy and Qi is plentiful, then Yin and Yang remain in balance. If the body becomes weakened, then it may be susceptible to damage by internal or external factors. In TCM the internal factors are the emotions, and the external factors are climatic conditions. Each organ is specially susceptible to certain of these (Fig. 8). The effects of the weather induce changes in the bodily climate similar to those seen in reality. Wind may produce movement and change; cold may cause tightness and contracture; damp may cause an accumulation of sticky fluids in the tissues. The emotions exist in all of us but, if excessive or unbalanced for prolonged periods, may produce profound pathological changes.

Fig. 8: Chart showing organ correspondences

ORGAN	EMOTION	CLIMATIC CONDITION
Lung	Grief and sadness	Dryness
Spleen	Depression and worry	Dampness
Heart	Joy	Heat
Kidney	Fear	Cold
Liver	Anger	Wind

The meridians and points

The meridians are distributed throughout the body, connecting the internal organs to the exterior surface. There are also fine linking meridians throughout the body that connect the channels, much as minor roads link major roads and form a network linking all areas not on the main routes. The meridians carry the Qi and blood to nourish the tissues, and they interweave within the body surface. They connect the organs to each other and the rest of the body, spreading their influence. If the defensive function is impaired or weakened, external pathogenic factors may invade and be transmitted deep into the body via the channels. Along these channels are places where the Qi is accessible at the surface and where it can be manipulated. Hundreds of these points have been identified and are used to affect the Qi of the meridian, its related organ and areas of influence.

There are 12 major meridians corresponding to the six Yin and six Yang organs. The Yang meridians lie on the posterior and lateral aspects of the trunk, head and limbs. Those assigned to Yin are found on the anterior aspect of the trunk and the medial aspects of the limbs. The connections of these channels link the Yin organs (Zang) to the Yang (Fu) and create a cyclical flow of Qi in the internally/externally paired meridians.

The meridians are named according to:

- The organ from which they arise
- Their Yin or Yang quality
- The limb of the body through which they run

The 12 major meridians

- The Lung Channel of Hand: Taiyin (Lu)
- The Large Intestine Channel of Hand: Yangming (LI)
- The Stomach Channel of Foot: Yangming (St)
- The Spleen Channel of Foot: Taiyin (Sp)
- The Heart Channel of Hand: Shaoyin (Ht)
- The Small Intestine Channel of Hand: Taiyang (SI)
- The Bladder Channel of Foot: Taiyang (Bl)
- The Kidney Channel of Foot: Shaoyin (Ki)
- The Heart Constrictor Channel of Hand: Jueyin (HC)
- The Triple Heater Channel of Hand: Shaoyang (TH)
- The Gall Bladder Channel of Foot: Shaoyang (GB)
- The Liver Channel of Foot: Jueyin (Li)

The last words in the above names describe the levels of Yin and Yang ascribed to the channels. The initials in parentheses are accepted abbreviations for the names, which will subsequently be used.

There are two other channels that have their own points. They run up the midline of the body: one posteriorly, the Du Channel (Yang), and one anteriorly, the Ren Channel (Yin). This gives a total of 14 meridians, from which points are selected for treatment.

The Yin Channels of Hand begin in their organs in the trunk and flow to the ends of the fingers, where they join the Yang Channels of Hand. These flow up to the head and connect to the Yang Channels of Foot. These run through the trunk to the toes, where they connect to the Yin Meridians of Foot. These flow up the legs and end in their organs in the body, completing the cycle. The Qi circulates through the meridians every 24 hours in the order shown in the diagram (Fig. 9).

Point location Accurate location of the points is necessary if treatment is to be effective. There are three main ways in which the positions of the points can be identified:

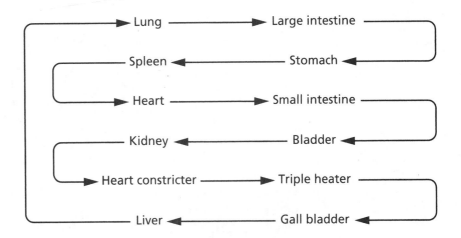

Fig. 9: Diagram to show the circulation of Qi

- Relationships to fixed anatomical structures
- Proportional distances
- Finger measurements

Many points lie near fixed structures, such as the sense organs, nipples, umbilicus, and so forth. Depressions and bony prominences are also useful landmarks. Proportional measuring is used on the limbs and trunk. A region is divided up into equal parts, and points are located by reference to these distances. Some of the major proportional divisions are shown in Figure 10. The unit of distance in these measurements is the *cun* or *tsun*. On the hand, 1 cun is equivalent to the width of the interphalangeal joint of the thumb, 3 cun to the width of the fingers at the level of the first interphalangeal joints. This of course depends on the patient's hands, as the distances are relative to each individual, although the therapist's hands can be used instead if his hands are a

Fig. 10: Major proportional divisions

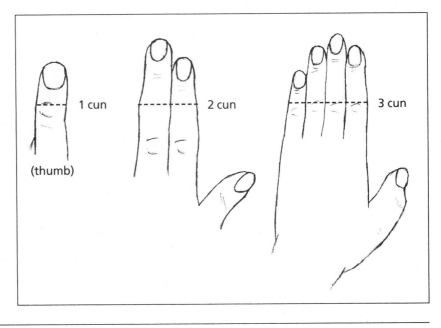

similar size. The easiest method is proportional division, the points being identified by splitting the distances into even fractions until the points are identified.

Once the point has been located by one of these methods, gentle palpation serves to identify the exact location. Sometimes the position can be felt as a small depression, or the skin may have a slightly different feel from the surrounding tissues. Whatever it feels like, differences can only be felt by light, subtle touching, and it is a skill that comes through practice and concentration. The points themselves are numbered to aid recognition and facilitate learning. The Yin Meridians of Hand (Lu, Ht, HC) begin in the body, so the numbers increase towards the end of the arm. The reverse is the case for the Yang Meridians of Hand (LI, TH, SI). These end at the head where they connect to the Yang Meridians of Foot (St, GB, Bl), whose numberings increase towards the feet. The numbers for the Yin Meridians of Foot (Ki, Sp, Li) start at the feet and increase towards the body.

Effects of acupressure

One of the primary effects is to improve the circulation of the blood. This in itself has a tonifying effect on the tissues. It also releases tension and spasm of the muscles, and can help to eliminate wastes from the muscles, so aiding recovery from fatigue. Acute and chronic pain can be eased by sedating treatments. Nerve conduction can be facilitated and the nerve tissue itself can be freed if it becomes limited by adhesions. Beneficial effects may also be seen in cases where there is over-activity in the nervous system. Calming, reducing treatments can bring about relaxation and reduce anxiety. Working on the body to bring it into a state of balance will also have a therapeutic effect on general health. This is because the proper flow of Qi in the channels affects the internal environment in a positive fashion. These physical effects are the result of treating the imbalances of Yin and Yang and Qi.

Principles of treatment

The aim of treatment is to balance Yin and Yang and to ensure the proper flow of Qi in the channels. Where the Qi is weak, it should be tonified, and where in excess, it should be calmed. If the flow of Qi becomes blocked or stagnant, it must be dispersed. As with all such treatments, how the practitioner relates to the patient is extremely important. Remain calm and focused throughout, and maintain a balanced posture that enables you to work without strain and tension. This will ensure that your own Qi will flow and allow you to help the movement of Qi in the patient. Concentrate on the effect you want, whether it be a calming or an invigorating effect. Do not treat if you are ill or unbalanced, as this may have an adverse effect on the patient's energy.

Pressure can be applied in several ways, depending on the required effect and the area of the body being treated. On large, flat areas, the pad of the thumb is used. Do not rest the body weight solely through the thumb as this may cause damage to the joints. Let the pressure be taken on the middle phalanx of the fingers, with the hand in a light fist. Points on the face and neck, and on the hands and feet, can be treated by 'nipping' with the tip or nail of the thumb or fingers. On large, fleshy areas, such as the hips and thighs, the elbows may be used, but care should be taken not to cause too much pain. For working along the channels, the palms or knuckles are useful. Allow the body to do the work. Do not hunch or tense the arms and shoulders, but stay relaxed and lean into the point to apply the pressure. This requires a balanced stance to allow you to move freely and control the pressure.

A good stance to use is to stand at an angle to the patient with the feet comfortably apart. Turn the front foot out by approximately 45 degrees and gently flex the knees. If you are working on the floor, ensure that you are in a comfortable position and support your weight between the arms and legs. This allows you to control the pressure and release it quickly if necessary. Do not carry on if you are uncomfortable – change your position before continuing. Tapping firmly with the tip of the index or middle finger along the channels and on the points is another way to activate the Qi. During all these treatments, sensations of soreness, tingling or distension may be felt by the patient. These sensations may be localized or felt along the course of the channels. This is a sign that the Qi of the channel is being activated and the prognosis is good. If no sensations are felt, it may be a sign that the Qi is very deficient or stuck. Regular treatment may be necessary to produce the desired effects. Do not confuse these sensations with pain. Heavy-handed pressure causing excessive discomfort will upset the patient and will not have a beneficial effect.

Working on the channels in the order of the circulation of Qi has an invigorating effect. Moving against the flow is said to have a reducing, calming effect. Light stimulation with movement is said to have a tonifying effect. Deeper, more sustained pressure has a reducing, sedating effect. When applying these deeper techniques, allow time for the tissues to release before moving down. Maintain the pressure for longer periods in this case. The intensity and duration of treatment will vary from patient to patient. In very deficient situations only extremely light, stimulating treatment will be tolerated. Over-treatment may cause the patient to become unwell or to faint. More robust types with excess conditions will require more vigorous treatment.

Using acupressure to treat

The cardinal signs of acute inflammation, heat, redness, pain and swelling show a Yang situation that requires calming. Western medicine recognizes this and uses the RICE procedure. This can be assisted by working on the channels around the area with reducing techniques. Local points can be selected or, if too tender and inflamed, points adjacent to the area. Ashi or tender points can also be treated. An additional advantage of acupressure in acute conditions is that, if the local area cannot be treated, then the points of that area on the other side of the body may be used with effect. This is especially useful if the injury has required some kind of protection, such as plaster. Muscle spasm is another Yang manifestation and this can likewise be treated.

The effect of these treatments is to increase venous and lymphatic drainage, reduce swelling and bleeding, and control pain and spasm. An acute situation may become chronic if it continues for some time. The pain may become a deep aching, and fibrous adhesions may begin to form. Muscles become stiff and local circulation poor, and the area becomes dysfunctional. This is an example of Qi and blood becoming blocked or stagnant in the channels. It is a Yang situation but may be due to an underlying deficiency. Treatment is aimed at dispersing the stagnation with reducing techniques and also at tonifying to treat the deficiency. Weakness and tightness of muscles can be due to a lack of Yang Qi and blood. This gives rise to a situation where the muscles are not adequately nourished and moistened and thus become stiff and inflexible. A tonifying treatment is indicated here to invigorate the circulation of Qi and blood. This will allow the muscles to soften and move. It may also be necessary to treat the opposing channels with reducing treatment if there is an imbalance. A good example of this may be seen in the spine. If the posture is slumped, with rounding of the back, this indicates weakness of Yang Qi in the Du channel. This runs up the centre of the spinal column and gives it support. An excess of energy in this channel may produce a tense, rigid spine that lacks flexibility. Treatment is aimed at balancing the Qi in the Ren and Du channels, so that the spine is supported but is also soft and flexible. That is why maintenance of good posture is so important.

Global weakness of muscles could indicate a problem with the spleen Zang function of nourishing the muscles or with circulation of Qi and blood. A hard, tight body might indicate a liver Zang disorder, where the smooth, harmonious flow of Qi in the muscles is impeded. In the former case, points could be selected on the stomach and spleen channels. The liver imbalance might require treatment of the liver and gall bladder channels.

Contraindications

There are relatively few contraindications to acupressure, but a few points need to be noted.

Avoid heavy pressure in osteoporotic patients. This is especially important on the spine and ribcage, but care should be taken in all areas. Deep sustained pressure should also be avoided on people who have delicate skin or who bruise easily. Open wounds or sores on the skin obviously should not be touched, to prevent infection. If the patient has recently had a serious illness or is very run down, do not treat excessively or for protracted periods. They may experience a feeling of unwellness or even fainting, due to their energy being very depleted. Treatment should also not be given if the patient has eaten a heavy meal recently.

There are several points that should not be treated in pregnancy: LI 4, Sp 6, Bl 60. Points on the abdomen should also be avoided, as should points in the lumbo-sacral area. In the latter stages of pregnancy, any points giving strong sensation must not be stimulated.

The point on the top of the head, Du 20, is not to be treated in those with high blood pressure. In cases of low blood pressure, Ki 1 on the sole of the foot should not be used.

As with all treatments, if any medical condition presents itself with which you are unfamiliar or about which you are unsure, do not treat, but seek advice from the patient's medical practitioner.

Common points in treatment

Below are some suggested points to use for problems in the areas of the neck and back, the shoulders, knees and ankles. It is by no means an exhaustive list, and you should attempt to become familiar with as many points as possible. The locations of the points mentioned are given in list form at the end of this chapter.

Points on the neck and back

Channels
The main channels involved in the back are the Du, bladder and gall bladder. In the neck, additionally, points on the Triple Heater and small intestine channels are used.

The back

Points
Select points in the relevant areas from the back Shu points on the bladder line. These are found 1.5 cun lateral to the spine, level with the lower borders of the tips of the spinous processes. For lateral problems use GB 30 and 34, and for central pain Du 4 and Shiqizhui (Extra), but do not use this if pain goes down the leg when pressed. Distal points on the bladder line are 54 and 60, especially if the pain is radiating down the back of the leg.

The neck

Points
Useful points here are GB 20 and 21, with Du 14 and Bl 11. SI 13 and 15 are also useful. If pain goes down the arm, select points on the relevant Channel of Hand. Common distal points are LI 4, SI 3 and TH 5. In addition, good effects are to be had by using GB 39 and Bl 60 on the leg.

The shoulders *Channels*
The main channels involved are the large intestine, small intestine and Triple Heater.

Points
Anteriorly, LI 15 is very important, also 14. TH 14 is used if the pain is more lateral. Posteriorly, SI 9, 10, 11 and 12, together with Du 14, have good effects on the shoulder. Distal points should be selected according to the involved channel. Common points are LI 11 and 4, SI 3 and TH 5.

The knees *Channels*
All of the Channels of Foot pass through the knee and points should be selected according to the location of the problem.

Points
Two Extra points are useful; called the Xiyan points, they lie on either side of the patellar tendon in the depressions found when the knee is flexed. The lateral Xiyan is also St 35. Other key points around the knee are St 36 (also an important point for general tonification) and GB 33 and 34. Medially, Sp 9 and 10 can be used, or Li 7 and 8. Posterior pain calls for Bl 53. Distally, Bl 60, GB 39, Sp 5 and Li 4 can be chosen.

The ankles *Channels*
All of the Channels of Foot may be affected here, and point selection is based on location of the problem.

Points
Laterally, points such as St 41, GB 39 and 40, and Bl 60 and 62 may be selected. Medially, Sp 5 and 6, Li 4 and Ki 3 can be of benefit.

This chapter has only touched on some of the principles of TCM. It is hoped that it will stimulate an interest in this different way of looking at health and disease. The most important thing is to become familiar with the concepts of TCM. Learn the positions and relationships of the channels, and build up a repertoire of points to use for common problems. If possible, attend a course to learn more about these arts.

Locations of the points Here are the locations of the points mentioned in the text (see recommended texts for further information).

LI 4	Between the thumb and index finger at the level of the mid-point of the first metacarpal
LI 11	With the elbow flexed, the point is located at the lateral end of the cubital crease

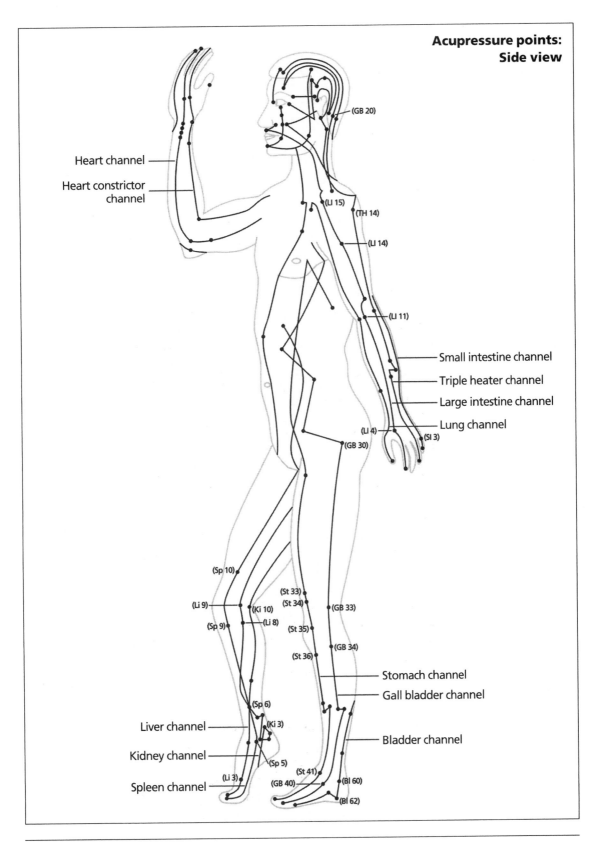

**Acupressure points:
Side view**

Heart channel

Heart constrictor
channel

(GB 20)

(LI 15)

(TH 14)

(LI 14)

(LI 11)

Small intestine channel

Triple heater channel

Large intestine channel

Lung channel

(LI 4)

(SI 3)

(GB 30)

(Sp 10)

(St 33)

(St 34)

(Li 9)

(Ki 10)

(GB 33)

(Sp 9)

(Li 8)

(St 35)

(GB 34)

(St 36)

Stomach channel

Gall bladder channel

(Sp 6)

Bladder channel

Liver channel

(Ki 3)

Kidney channel

(Sp 5)

(St 41)

Spleen channel

(Li 3)

(GB 40)

(Bl 60)

(Bl 62)

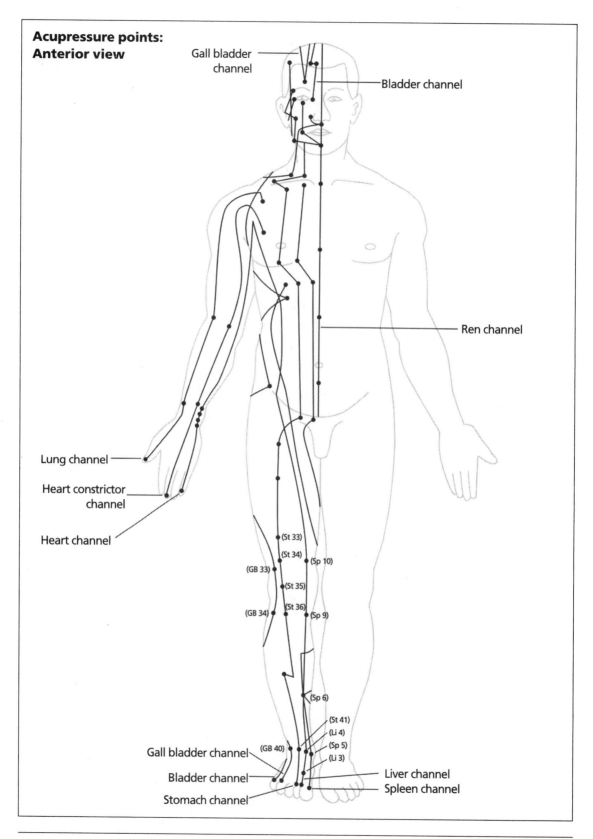

Acupressure points: Anterior view

Gall bladder channel

Bladder channel

Ren channel

Lung channel

Heart constrictor channel

Heart channel

(St 33)

(St 34)

(Sp 10)

(GB 33)

(St 35)

(GB 34)

(St 36)

(Sp 9)

(Sp 6)

(St 41)

(Li 4)

(Sp 5)

(Li 3)

Gall bladder channel

(GB 40)

Liver channel

Bladder channel

Spleen channel

Stomach channel

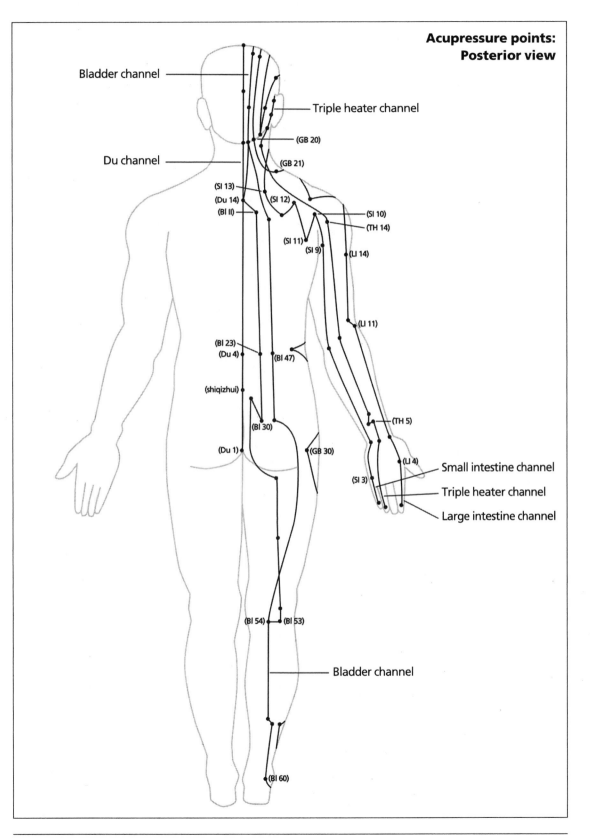

Acupressure points: Posterior view

Bladder channel

Triple heater channel

(GB 20)

Du channel

(GB 21)

(SI 13)
(Du 14)
(BI II)

(SI 12)

(SI 10)
(TH 14)

(SI 11)
(SI 9)

(LI 14)

(LI 11)

(BI 23)
(Du 4)

(BI 47)

(shiqizhui)

(BI 30)

(TH 5)

(Du 1)

(GB 30)

(LI 4)

(SI 3)

Small intestine channel

Triple heater channel

Large intestine channel

(BI 54) (BI 53)

Bladder channel

(BI 60)

LI 14	Just above the lower insertion of the deltoid in the midline of the arm
LI 15	With the arm abducted, the point is located in the anterior depression on the deltoid muscle just below the acromion
TH 5	2 cun above the posterior crease of the wrist between the radius and ulna
TH 14	At the level of LI 15 in the posterior depression when the arm is abducted
SI 3	Proximal to the 5th metacarpal joint at the junction of the red and white skin when a loose fist is made
SI 9	With the arm at the side, the point is 1 cun above the posterior end of the axillary fold on the posterior aspect of the shoulder joint
SI 10	Directly above SI 9 in the depression below the lateral end of the spine of the scapula
SI 11	In the middle of the scapula below the spine, two-thirds of the distance up from the inferior angle
SI 12	Above SI 11 in the midpoint of the suprascapular fossa (abduct the arm, and the point is in the depression)
SI 13	On the medial extremity of the superior scapular fossa (midway between SI 10 and the spinous process of T2)
SI 15	2 cun lateral to Du 14
St 33	With the knee flexed, on a line from the anterior superior iliac spine to the patella, 3 cun above the lateral superior border of the patella
St 34	With the knee flexed, 2 cun above the lateral superior border of the patella
St 36	3 cun below ST 35 (lateral Xiyan), 1 finger breadth lateral to the anterior crescent of the tibia
St 41	On the dorsum of the foot at the midpoint of the transverse crease of the ankle joint, in the depression between the extensor digitorum longus and the hallucis longus, at the level of the tip of the external malleolus
Sp 5	In the depression distal and inferior to the medial malleolus, midway between the tuberosity of the navicular and the tip of the medial malleolus
Sp 6	3 cun above the tip of the medial malleolus on the posterior border of the tibia
Sp 9	On the lower border of the medial condyle of the tibia, in the depression on the medial border of the tibia
Sp 10	With the knee flexed, the point is 2 cun above the medial superior border of the patella on the bulge of the vastus medialis
Bl 11	1.5 cun lateral to the lower border of the tip of the spinous process of T1

Back Shu	Points found on the Bl line 1.5 cun lateral to the lower borders of the tips of the spinous processes of the vertebrae down to L5
Bl 53	Lateral to Bl 54 on the medial border of the biceps femoris
Bl 54	Midpoint of the popliteal crease at the back of the knee
Bl 60	In the depression between the lateral malleolus and the tendo-Achilles at the ankle
Bl 62	In the depression directly below the tip of the lateral malleolus
Ki 3	In the depression between the tendo-Achilles and the tip of the medial malleolus
GB 20	Lateral to the occiput at the level of DU 16
GB 21	Midway between Du 14 and the acromion in the upper fibres of the trapezius
GB 30	Side-lying hip-flexed, divide the distance between the sacral hiatus and the great trochanter of the hip into three parts. The point lies at the junction of the lateral and middle thirds
GB 33	3 cun above GB 34 between the biceps femoris and the femur
GB 34	In the hollow anterior and inferior to the head of the fibula
GB 39	3 cun above the lateral malleolus on the anterior border of the fibula
GB 40	Anterior and inferior to the lateral malleolus in the depression lateral to the extensor digitorum longus
Li 3	Between the 1st and 2nd metatarsals at the proximal junction of the two bones
Li 4	1 cun anterior to the medial malleolus between the extensor hallucis longus and the tibialis anterior (midway between ST 41 and Sp 5)
Li 7	In the medial head of the gastrocnemius, 1 cun posterior to Sp 9
Li 8	With the knee flexed, the point lies at the medial end of the crease, anterior to the semimembranosus and semitendinosus
Du 4	Between L2 and L3 spinous processes in the midline of the spine
Du 14	Just below the spinous process of C7 in the midline

Extra points

Shiqizhui	Just below the 5th lumbar spinous process in the midline
Xiyan points	2 points, one medial, one lateral, in the depressions on either side of the patellar tendon at the knee

16 Remedial Exercise

When treating musculoskeletal problems, the therapist should first assess the patient to determine the muscles that are weak and those that are excessively tight. Occasionally injury occurs because muscles are too strong or too flexible, but these are far less common occurrences. When performing massage treatment, the tissues are palpated by the therapist very thoroughly, which can give him an even more detailed understanding of the exact location of weakness and tension.

At the end of massage treatment, the situation should be re-assessed to see what improvement has taken place and how much of the problem remains. Sometimes a full recovery may appear to have occurred, but realistically the therapist should consider the possibility that some of the symptoms may return. Even when a patient has a general massage, without the presence of a specific injury, areas of tension and weakness may still be identified. These could be the sites of potential injury in the future, or they may be adversely affecting function and general well-being, without the patient being aware of it.

Whatever the situation, remedial exercises to stretch out tension and improve strength will add greatly to the effect of the treatment. Immediately after massage the muscles are warm and relaxed, and they will respond extremely well to remedial exercises applied by the therapist. If similar exercises are also performed regularly by the patient afterwards, then the beneficial effects of the treatment may continue to take place indefinitely. Where the patient is undergoing a course of treatment, this also means that the therapist is more able to make continual progress, with less regression between sessions.

Of the two situations, tension and weakness, it is important to deal with the tight areas first. These restrict movement and may also inhibit nerve stimulation to weaker opposing muscles, making it difficult to exercise and strengthen them effectively. Often just releasing tension will improve function and allow the weak areas to strengthen up naturally through more normal use.

Stretching

Developing good stretching techniques is perhaps as much an art as it is a science, as there are so many variables involved. A therapist who is new to this subject should start by developing and practising a range of standard stretches for all the main muscles and groups. Then many variations can be developed from them as experience grows.

There are a great number of muscles, both large and small, all of which have a specific function. So an individual muscle needs to be carefully isolated by positioning and fixing the patient so that the stretch is focused through it. With the muscles that work one joint only, this is usually quite simple, but with two-joint (or more) muscles it becomes more complicated. One joint needs to be fixed so that it pre-stretches the muscle, while the other joint is moved to increase the stretch. This means that there may be two different techniques for the same muscle to focus the stretch at either end.

General stretches for a muscle or group will release tension generally throughout the area. But specific problems often only affect a small part of the muscle, and a general stretch may be accommodated by the healthy tissues without the specific part being affected. Within each stretch there needs to be some 'fine tuning', by careful adjustments in the position, to try and focus the stretch into the target area. This can be made easier if deep massage has already been applied, as the patient will have been made aware of the exact location of the problem, and can tell the therapist when he feels the stretch in the same place.

Muscle length and flexibility can vary greatly between individuals, because of injury, general conditioning and hereditary factors. A position that may cause a maximal stretch in one patient may produce no stretch at all in another. Different holding positions need to be developed, which take account of the individual starting point that will best suit the patient. Different positions also need to be developed to adapt to practical and environmental factors; stretches may need to be done standing or sitting, at the work-place or at an outdoor sports event, etc.

The muscle must be fully relaxed and non-weight-bearing, otherwise it will not stretch fully, even though the patient may still feel a sensation of stretch. To help achieve this, the quality of the therapist's handling skill is vital and needs good contact and firm support. It is important to get verbal feedback from the patient to be sure that the stretch is felt in the right place. This will also improve the patient's self-awareness and will make it more likely that he does the stretch correctly when he performs it himself.

When stretching a muscle, it should first be taken slowly to the point where the patient feels a mild discomfort, and then it should be held firmly but comfortably in that position. No sensation of actual pain, tearing or burning should be felt, as this would suggest that the fibres are being over-stretched and torn. After a period of time (from 10 seconds upwards) the tissues may begin to ease and the stretch can be gently increased. There are many differing opinions as to how long a stretch should be held, but it is generally accepted that the length of time is more significant than the intensity of the stretch. Short ballistic-type stretches or using too much force can increase tension through a reflex action. Long, sustained and progressive stretching (for up to 90 seconds or even longer) seems to produce the best results (see MET in Chapter 14).

Strengthening

Isolating the action of a specific muscle so that it can actively be strengthened can present similar problems to stretching. The difficulty arises because if a muscle (or part of it) becomes weak, movement patterns instinctively alter slightly, so other muscles take up the load. Without careful control of the movement to prevent this, the strong muscles will be strengthened further and the weak area will remain unaffected. Muscles can be strengthened in a variety of ways:

Active movements The patient actively contracts the muscle through its fullest range of movement, without any resistance or loading. This is necessary after acute injury and helps restore function rather than real strength, but it is a vital first step in rehabilitation. The range and control of movement are the primary concern, so movement should begin very slowly, with the patient being encouraged to move as far as possible.

Isometric contraction The muscle is fixed at a certain position along its range and the patient contracts against a fixed resistance, without any actual movement taking place. This is particularly useful in maintaining strength in a muscle that cannot be exercised normally, due to dysfunction in its associated joint. The strengthening effect is greatest in the middle and inner range of movement. Isometric contraction increases intramuscular pressure, which can compress blood vessels and reduce the oxygen supply to the cells, so it should not be applied for more than about 10 seconds at a time. (Due to the compression of blood vessels, it may be contraindicated in some medical conditions.)

Concentric movements This is the most common type of muscle-strengthening activity and involves the contraction and shortening of a muscle by taking it through its active range of movement with a weighted resistance. For example, the biceps muscle concentrically contracts when lifting a weight, by flexing the elbow.

A muscle produces its greatest force in the mid-range, and if heavy weights are used, the patient may only be able to use this part of the range and is likely to assist the overall movement with other muscles. If the muscle is only trained in the mid-range, it will only function in that range and may become chronically short. Although heavy weights may need to be used to restore balance with other powerful muscles, it is important always to include exercises with light resistance through the fullest range to develop length as well.

The movements should also be made slowly to develop control throughout the range. Sudden, quick contractions can lead to injury and are likely to increase muscle tension by over-stimulating the nerve receptors (golgi tendon organs). As momentum accounts for much of the movement, the muscle will not develop strength through its inner range either.

Eccentric movements

This involves the muscles starting in the inner range and contracting against a greater resistance, which forces the muscle to extend, even though the fibres themselves are shortening. For example, the biceps eccentrically contracts when lowering a weight slowly with the elbow extending. This is the most powerful way of strengthening a muscle, but it is more likely to cause the fibres to tear if too great a force is used, so it should not be used in the early recovery stage of an injury.

With the fibres contracting but the muscle lengthening, a considerable shearing force takes place between the actual fibres. This breaks fibrous adhesions and releases tension, making it a good technique for long-term chronic problems.

Isokinetic movements

In this type of exercise, the muscle contracts through its full range at a constant speed and the resistance varies according to the muscle's capability. Where the power of the muscle is greatest, in the mid-range, the resistance is highest, and through the inner and outer ranges it is reduced. This method is only possible with sophisticated specialist equipment, but on an intuitive level a therapist can often achieve much the same effect using 'hands-on' resistance. The great advantage of isokinetic training is that it can produce maximum strength throughout the maximum range. Unfortunately, the equipment is not readily available and the technique is very labour-intensive for the therapist to perform.

Functional exercises

Muscle imbalance often leads to an alteration in a functional movement pattern, as the body instinctively learns to compensate for the problem. Over a period of time the nervous system accepts this as a normal pattern, and restoring muscle balance alone may not change this. If the faulty pattern continues, the imbalance and injury are very likely to return.

As well as restoring local muscle balance with stretching and strengthening exercises, it is vital that more functional exercises should also be performed to restore good movement patterns. This can normally be done by making carefully controlled movements that imitate normal everyday actions, often using just a light resistance. The patient will instinctively want to use the poor pattern, which feels more natural, so the therapist must carefully observe the movement and get the patient to make corrections where necessary. The patient should be made to focus on the feeling of the movement pattern and, if necessary, should use a mirror to observe the movement when doing these exercises on his own.

These functional exercises will also improve co-ordination and proprioception, which are particularly important in the weight-bearing joints involved in walking and running. Along with any soft tissue damage, the nervous system is also disrupted, which can result in joint instability. Without restoring good proprioceptive function through balancing exercises, injury is likely to recur, even though the muscles' strength may be fully restored.

Functional integrity Postural and functional restrictions in one part of the body may not cause painful symptoms locally but can lead to over-use and injury in other parts. It is often necessary to consider the functional integration of all parts of the body to find distant areas of restriction that may be causing a local problem.

Example 1

Restricted movement in the lumbar spine can lead to over-use and injury in the vertebral joint areas above and below it, as they have to make up for the deficiency. Often this lumbar restriction builds up over many years, and when the patient is asked to make independent flexion and extension movements in just the lumbar spine, by tilting the pelvis forward and back, he sometimes find it impossible to do so. As well as physical difficulty due to tension in the tissue, on a neuromuscular level he may find it difficult actually to create this movement.

The therapist should help and encourage the patient to do this exercise correctly, without any other body movement occurring. At first only a few degrees of movement may be possible, but the patient should focus on the feeling and experience of this action to create better functional awareness. Eventually the range will increase and, with greater awareness, the patient may naturally use more lumbar mobility during normal activities and so reduce the likelihood of over-using other parts.

Example 2

Restriction in the shoulder girdle often leads to over-use injury at the shoulder joint or neck area. To improve mobility here, the patient can sit with his hands resting palm upwards on his lap. Without moving the arm, neck or shoulder joint itself, he should attempt to make slow movements with the shoulder girdle only. Concentrating on maximum range, separate movements should be made up and down, backwards and forwards, as well as circling in both directions. Again the patient should concentrate on the feeling of these movements to improve functional awareness so that they can become a more natural part of all neck and shoulder actions.

Compliance It is important to recommend exercises that the patient can do himself to promote recovery and improve general well-being. This not only has a therapeutic value but can also have a strong psychological effect.

Instead of feeling like the passive victim of an injury and dependent on the therapist, he becomes actively involved in his own recovery. Patients commonly ask (usually in the first five minutes of their visit) how soon they can get back to normal activity. But this is often an impossible question for the therapist to answer, as so many other factors are involved. If a patient with a knee injury has a sedentary occupation, which allows plenty of rest, it will probably recover much more quickly than that of a patient who has to climb up and down stairs all day. With remedial exercise, the patient can make comparisons with the other side of his body (in the case of a limb), and can monitor his own rate of recovery.

But, as with massage treatment itself, there is no standard set of techniques that will suit all patients. Exercises need to be found that are not only effective but, more importantly, are ones that the patient will actually do (the compliance factor). People who do not normally do any formal sport or exercise are unlikely to maintain a programme that takes too much time, requires space and involves a number of repetitions and levels of effort. This will not fit easily into their lifestyle, they may not properly understand what is required and they are unlikely to perform the exercises correctly without supervision. Instead, such patients should be recommended simple exercises that can be done without great formality, at the work-place, while they are on the telephone, running the bath or boiling the kettle, etc. They are much more likely to do these exercises, which can occasionally act as a catalyst, making the patient more physically aware of his body and developing a more active interest in his own well-being.

When treating a patient who is involved in a particular sport or exercise, a more formal programme can be offered, but again it must be suited to the individual. Consider first the exercises normally carried out, in detail, and then recommend changes according to the specific needs of the condition. Certain exercises may need to be omitted if they could be aggravating the problem, while others may need to be altered or improved, and new ones added. The most important consideration is that the exercises must fit in with what the patient normally does, otherwise the compliance factor will be poor.

To do this successfully, the therapist needs to develop a broad understanding of many types of exercise: the numerous styles of aerobics classes, modern gym equipment, athletic training (intervals, repetitions, hill sessions, etc.), yoga, dance, to name but a few.

Communication Communication is another factor that can affect compliance. Up to 50 per cent of information is forgotten after just five minutes and a further 25 per cent is forgotten almost immediately after the session. The more information the patient is given, the more he will forget, so clear but brief instructions are better than lengthy explanations. This also means that it may be better to recommend a few exercises initially, to get the patient started, and then build on this at following sessions. It is also common for patients to misunderstand instructions, even though they usually nod and say 'yes' enthusiastically, and it is hard for the therapist to realize this. It may help to get the patient to repeat the instructions and demonstrate the exercises before they leave.

A patient is more likely to comply correctly with instructions if he has a good understanding of the problem. As has already been shown, verbal communication has a big wastage factor, so visual and tactile means should also be used. Wall charts of the muscular and skeletal systems can be used to show the tissues involved, and can help the patient to visualize the situation and see why the exercises will be of benefit. And, as explained earlier, by palpation of the tissues involved and by feeling the exercises being performed, the patient can also be made more self-aware.

One other very important factor is the personal way in which the therapist deals with the patient. Despite all the technical skills that the therapist may have to offer, it is the quality of the one-to-one relationship that often produces the strongest response. Massage treatment takes time and individual attention, which in the busy modern world is a rare commodity, and this is greatly valued by the patient. To take full advantage of this situation, the therapist should prevent any outside distractions so that the patient has his full attention. He should also show empathy, interest and concern for the patient's overall well-being, and not just for the injury or problem being treated.

17 Massage with Medical Conditions

Massage should never be considered as a method of diagnosing or treating medical conditions, as this should always be the responsibility of a medical practitioner. In a complementary role, however, massage has much to offer patients suffering from a very wide variety of medical complaints.

As massage stimulates the circulation, it promotes the healing process and, providing it is safe to use it, will always have some therapeutic benefit. The good psychological effects often achieved through massage can also have a positive effect on recovery and can sometimes lead to quite remarkable results.

This book does not explain the physiology of medical conditions in any great detail. The therapist must use other sources to study the systems of the body and to learn how they function and dysfunction. When dealing with any medical condition it is most important to know if there are any contraindications to massage relating either to the locally affected area or to the body as a whole. If you have a clear diagnosis from a doctor and an understanding of the relevant pathology, then the efficacy and possible uses of massage can be determined. Even with conditions that are safe to treat, it is necessary to know the patient's past medical history, as this may raise other considerations. If there is any doubt about this most important subject, consult the patient's doctor before treating.

In very general terms, any organ or tissue that is *inflamed* for any reason is contraindicated for local massage. *Infections* are usually contraindicated for general treatment, as they could increase the inflammation, spreading it to other areas, and cause the patient considerable pain. In the post-acute, recovery or chronic phase of these conditions, massage may often become possible, and indeed beneficial, in promoting recovery. But just when a condition becomes safe to treat is sometimes difficult to judge. Whenever there is some doubt, the first treatment should be carried out very cautiously, with light techniques for only a short time. The patient's response should then be checked over the next few days, before treating again.

When treating soft tissue injuries, some techniques may cause considerable pain but still be safe and effective, but this is never the case when treating people with medical complaints. Mild discomfort may be acceptable but if actual pain is caused while giving massage, then the treatment should be stopped and the patient's doctor informed.

This chapter outlines some of the uses of massage for situations affecting various systems of the body and also for some particular common conditions. It is not intended as a comprehensive guide but rather as an outline of the possibilities. The therapist should consider each patient as an individual and develop a treatment approach accordingly.

Respiratory system

The common features of respiratory conditions are a difficulty in breathing and/or coughing, both of which involve considerable muscle activity. These muscles can suffer over-use and micro-trauma in the same way as any other muscle and can cause painful symptoms and increased tension. This could add to the patient's discomfort and increase their breathing difficulties. In the long term, even when the patient has recovered from the condition, chronic muscle tension may continue to restrict breathing and predispose the patient to other respiratory problems. With permanent chronic conditions, like asthma or bronchitis, posture can eventually become affected, with the shoulders raised, a hollow chest and a rounded (kyphotic) thoracic spine. Again, this can further increase the patient's difficulties.

Massage can be beneficial in all these situations by attending to damaged, fatigued and tightened muscles. It can also produce general relaxation and greater structural freedom.

Over the chest area, as well as effleurage and petrissage techniques, deep stroking and friction can be applied to the intercostal and subclavicular muscles, which often become tense and fibrous. With women it is not possible to do this through the breast tissue, but working through a towel it is possible to apply deep pressure through one finger in the space between the sterno/costal joints and thereby achieve a neuromuscular effect along the whole intercostal section. Friction/pressure on an intercostal muscle combined with deep inhalation achieves a good Soft Tissue Release effect.

It is also important to treat the abdomen area, because muscle contraction here creates the internal pressure that assists the diaphragm in forced exhalation and coughing. Tension can increase over a period of time and the muscles may become less able to assist respiration. The diaphragm can similarly be affected and friction can reach the anterior fibres of this muscle (see p.126) and can be highly effective.

The muscles of the back and the ligaments around the spine should also be treated, as tension can build up here too. The thoracic spine needs to function freely to assist the breathing process. Massage to this area will also benefit the spinal nerves, which supply the respiratory organs as well as the musculature.

Patients will often find it difficult (or have a greater need) to clear their lungs of excess fluid. To some extent this can be assisted by percussion techniques, applied slightly more heavily than normal, over the back and chest. (Other physiotherapy techniques to assist in clearing the lungs should only be carried out by someone properly trained to do so.)

With chronic, long-term conditions, posture and muscle balance can become permanently affected. Massage alone may not be enough to prevent this, and the patient needs to exercise in order to prevent the problem.

Strengthen weakened or stretched muscles: usually the rhomboids and latissimus dorsi. Stretch tight muscles: usually the pectorals and upper trapezius. (Many other muscles – serratus, abdominals, etc. – may also need to be considered, depending on the individual.)

Breathing and mobility exercises for the neck, shoulders and back will be beneficial and should be encouraged.

Some respiratory conditions, like asthma, can be stress-related, and in other conditions the breathing difficulties themselves can be a stressful experience. Regular massage treatment to promote relaxation, with advice on relaxation and deep breathing exercises, can greatly help the patient cope with his situation.

Nervous system

General   There are many conditions of the nervous system, affecting all parts: the brain, spinal chord or the peripheral network. The common feature, from the massage therapist's point of view, is that most conditions have an effect on the nerve conductivity to skeletal muscles. Where this occurs only in the sensory (afferent) network, muscle function will not be affected and the benefit of massage will be simply in assisting the general health of the area. The feeling that a patient experiences during massage, particularly during tapotement (percussion), can sometimes stimulate nerve response and so may help their actual condition.

Where the motor nerves are affected, dysfunction will develop in the muscles (and organs) that they serve. Although treating the muscles may not have any direct therapeutic effect on the nerve itself, by improving the condition of the muscles, the actual dysfunction may not be as great.

The most common symptom is muscle weakness, or wasting, due to a reduction in nerve stimulation, and the muscle becomes hypotonic. Due to reduced muscle activity, blood circulation in the area may be poor and massage can help this and improve the general health of the tissues, and so too their function. Vigorous tapotement can stimulate the nerve receptors and improve muscle tone, so helping to improve the condition, too.

Sometimes muscles may become excessively tense (hypertonic) or go into spasm due to over-stimulation. Deep stroking techniques can have a beneficial stretching effect and help release this tension. Tapotement, however, should not be used on these muscles, as it stimulates and so may further increase tension.

Massage treatment to the area of dysfunction attends only to the symptoms; improvement in function requires the patient's effort (and effective medical treatment of the root cause). It is necessary to exercise to strengthen weak muscles and stretch tense ones. Remember that it is important to release tight muscles first, otherwise they could reciprocally inhibit nerve supply to the weak ones, which will prevent them from strengthening.

The functional effect of nerve conditions may not just be apparent with gross general movements, for it is often the control of movement that is most affected. An exercise programme should include some movement patterns (without weights) that require control and should be done as slowly and smoothly as possible.

Neuralgia   This is caused by the compression or tethering of a nerve as it passes through or between other tissues, and tends to occur if these are swollen, damaged or congested with scar tissue. The compression may restrict nerve impulses, and a tethering can prevent the nerve from stretching out sufficiently to accommodate body movements. Either way the soft tissues (or organs) that the nerves supply can become affected.

Symptoms may not be apparent at the site of the problem itself, and may only be felt in the referred area further along the nerve. Treatment of the symptom area will have no effect on the actual condition itself. By tracing back along the path of the nerve, using deep stroking and friction techniques, it is sometimes possible to identify and treat the site of the compression or tethering. This tends to be a point where the nerve passes along a groove or tunnel in the bone, usually at a joint. Scar tissue in such a confined space can cause the impingement (for example, carpal tunnel syndrome in the wrist). Friction can break this down and free the nerve, as well as stimulating the circulation to aid its recovery.

Where nerve entrapment occurs at a joint, particularly between two vertebrae (a common secondary symptom in spondylosis and ankylosing spondylitis), massage may sometimes be of benefit in a secondary way. By releasing the soft tissues around the spine and increasing freedom of movement, pressure may be taken off the nerve.

Neuritis   This is caused by inflammation of the nerve (usually to its sheath or connective tissue) and the symptoms tend to be much the same as for neuralgia, though it tends to ache more but cause less dysfunction. The inflamed nerve usually lies deep within the body, so general massage and light friction are beneficial, with little risk of aggravating the problem. After the inflammation has gone, the tissues around the nerve may be thick and fibrous which may lead to neuralgia. They should be treated with deep friction.

Sciatica This is the common name given to any condition that results in disrupted function through the sciatic nerve, and can be caused by either neuralgia (which is more common) or neuritis. Nerve entrapment usually occurs in front of the sacroiliac joint, beneath the piriformis, beneath the gluteus maximus, over the quadratus femoris and obturator internus or between the hamstrings. Disruption to any of the lumbar and sacral vertebrae may also cause entrapment. Referred motor and/or sensory symptoms can be experienced in any tissues along the leg, but treating those sites alone will have no effect.

Due to the deep location of the problem, it is often difficult to treat sciatica with massage (and impossible in front of the sacroiliac), but if deep friction is possible, then the results can be excellent. The muscles of the lower back, hips and hamstrings need to be softened first as much as possible with general massage techniques. To locate and treat the area of damage it is best to try a variety of side-lying, hip-flexed positions to enable palpation of the deep tissues of the lower back and hip from different angles and directions. When deep friction is applied to the right area it often creates the referred symptoms. If these go away within a few seconds after releasing the pressure, then it is safe to continue. If they continue for some time, this suggests that the nerve is inflamed, and treatment may continue but more gently, to prevent causing the symptomatic pain.

A similar scenario can occur to the brachial nerve, which supplies the arm (brachial neuralgia). Treatment procedures are the same as with neuralgia and sciatica, but arthritic conditions are also more likely to be involved here.

Abdomen and viscera conditions

General In the acute phase these will all be contraindicated, but in many post-acute or chronic conditions abdomen massage can be beneficial. It will not only help the muscles, releasing tension and improving tone and function, but will also improve peristaltic activity and the flow of substances through the intestines. The smooth muscle that makes up the walls of the intestines will respond to massage in much the same way as the striated skeletal muscle, and so its function too can be improved. Long-term chronic problems can result in areas of fibrosis and adhesions developing in any of the visceral tissues, and this can be broken down with the careful use of friction. Massage also stimulates circulation and the flow of interstitial fluids, which is another benefit that is of great importance in this area.

Many abdominal conditions, such as colitis and irritable bowel syndrome, are believed to have a stress-related component. Not only can massage help the symptoms of these conditions, but it can do much to address the stress aspect as well.

Chronic complaints affecting particular organs such as the liver may benefit from the stimulation of blood-flow through massage. After general abdominal work to soften the superficial muscles, deep petrissage techniques can be used over particular organs to good effect.

Constipation Blockages in the intestines will cause poor digestion and can sometimes be felt as a small, hard lump. This can be treated with massage, providing it is a simple blockage with no underlying factors to consider. Gentle friction should be applied to the specific area with deep stroking away from it, to loosen and help move it along.

Where a blockage occurs in the large intestine, this will cause constipation. Subject to other factors, massage can be an effective form of treatment and, with minor conditions, may be preferable to oral medication. First it is necessary to work on the large intestine from the blockage in a clockwise direction, through the descending colon using deep stroking techniques. This clears any congestion ahead of the problem and improves the chances of success. Then light friction can be applied to the blockage in an effort to break it down, so that it can pass freely along the system. Stroking techniques must not be applied up the ascending colon and towards the blockage, as this could increase the congestion and so worsen the problem.

Great care must be taken not to over-treat this condition in a single session. Too much friction may cause inflammation of the colon, which must be avoided at all costs.

Arthritis

Arthritis is the common name given to a number of different chronic degenerative joint conditions. Millions of people are affected by it and any therapist will undoubtedly get patients who say they have 'a bit of arthritis'. Quite often they will not know what type of arthritis it is, and may not even have consulted a doctor about it. Even when it has been medically diagnosed, it is such a common condition that physiotherapy cannot be made available to all sufferers. Oral medication is often the only course of treatment offered to patients, which if taken for very long periods can have other side-effects. Physiotherapy is often only given in advanced stages of the condition, when it may too late to make much improvement. So there is considerable scope for massage therapy to help in the control and management of this painful and debilitating condition.

Osteoarthritis (OA) This condition affects individual joints and is usually due to excessive wear and tear or a past traumatic injury. It is therefore more common in weight-bearing joints like the hip, knee, lumbar and lower cervical spine, as well as the joints of the hand. Excessive use does not, however, automatically mean that OA will occur; marathon runners, for example, do not appear to be more likely to suffer from OA in the hip in later life than sedentary people.

The first structure affected is the articular cartilage, which becomes more fibrous and eventually wears away at the point of greatest pressure. This allows the bones to rub together and the surfaces become hard and polished. As this occurs, debris collects around the margins of this polished area, which can calcify and roughen the surface, causing further damage as well as restricting joint movement.

The soft tissues around the joint become affected as a result of the chronic inflammation within it. The synovial capsule and surrounding ligaments may thicken and become inflamed, and occasionally pieces may flake off and become loose bodies floating around in the joint capsule. If these loose bodies become lodged between structures like the articulating bones, then there can be severe joint restriction.

Pain usually comes on gradually and in the early stages there may not be any visible swelling or redness, although later on the joint can become very swollen and eventually even deformed. Pain is often felt most when the joint is kept immobile, or when weight-bearing, and stiffness is normally worse in the morning. A creaking sensation (crepitus) may also be experienced.

The development of pain and restriction in the joint's range leads to less activity and subsequent wastage in the associated muscles. As the muscles become weaker, the patient becomes less able to work the joint properly and so the stiffness is further increased, and so on.

Treatment

General massage techniques to improve the condition of the muscles of an affected joint can help its function. With better function and use, calcification and fibrosis are less able to form, which helps prevent further degenerative changes. Due to limited joint range, it may not be possible to perform good stretching exercises, so some muscles may become excessively tight, and deep stroking techniques can be an effective way of releasing this tension.

The chronic inflammation in OA will not normally be aggravated by massage, as it occurs at the articular surface deep within the joint, where direct treatment cannot reach. Providing the soft tissues around the joint are not also inflamed, they can be treated with all massage techniques including friction, which will break down scar tissue and fibrous adhesions as well as improving joint lubrication.

Active and resisted exercises within the pain-free range should be encouraged to maintain good muscle function. Passive movements can be applied very gently to try to increase range, but these should be carried out under medical supervision whenever possible.

Spondylosis This is a degenerative condition, similar to OA, which affects the intervertebral joints and is associated with the wear and tear commonly caused by postural and occupational stress. The joints normally affected are C4 to T1 (leading to a deformity known as 'Dowager's hump'), T4 to T6 and L2 to L4, although other parts of the spine can also be affected as they compensate for the problem.

As bad posture and movement patterns help cause the condition, there is obviously a considerable soft tissue factor involved. Not only does chronic muscle tension and imbalance help bring on the condition, but as arthritic changes take place in the joints the muscles become further affected by this. The ligaments around the joint also become thicker and less pliable.

Exercises to improve posture and movement are vital to control spondylosis, but if the muscles are in poor condition it may be impossible to do this effectively. Deep massage and friction to loosen tense areas, especially around the vertebrae (unless acute), are essential to enable the patient to carry out the exercises needed to manage the condition. As well as the affected joint, it is important to work deeply around the sections of the spine above and below it, as good function there may help take some of the load off the damaged joints.

Rheumatoid arthritis (RA) This is a condition that is still not well understood, but although the actual cause is unknown, it is believed to relate to a malfunction of the auto-immune system. It tends to affect the same joints on both sides of the body and is most common in the hand, elbow, shoulder, foot and knee.

The development of the disease is variable, but there tend to be sporadic periods of acute inflammation with periods of remission in between. Unlike OA, where the condition starts deep within the joint and moves outward, RA begins in the outer tissues and progresses inwards. The first structure to be affected is the synovial capsule, which, it is believed, is attacked by the immune system as though it were a foreign body, which causes it to become acutely inflamed.

As the capsule is affected, any joint movement will be painful, and as it becomes swollen there can be intense aching, even when immobile. Rest is essential and ice packs may ease the discomfort, but massage treatment of the joint itself is contraindicated during the acute inflammation period.

When the condition goes into remission, the capsule may remain thicker and more fibrous, and permanent creases can form in the outer membrane, which will affect the range of movement. Secretion of synovial fluid may be excessive and watery at first, but later on becomes thicker and further stiffens the joint. After repeated inflammatory periods, the tissue damage progresses into the joint and eventually affects the articular cartilage. It then takes on the characteristics of OA as well, eventually leading to severe deformity that may need replacement surgery.

The immobility and need for rest during inflamed periods, and the progressive restriction in movement during remissions, have their effect on the associated muscles. Weakness and atrophy are the main problems, but tension can also build up, due to the inability of the joint to allow them to stretch. RA can affect the connective tissue, making it thick and less porous, which also adversely affects the muscle. As with OA, poor muscle tone affects joint function, which further affects the muscles, and so on.

Treatment

While mysteries remain about the cause of RA there will be some debate about the safe use of massage. During periods of acute inflammation the joint cannot be treated, but is it safe to apply massage to other areas? Stroking techniques away from the inflamed joint to reduce swelling may possibly also help spread the disease to other joints. RA is extremely common in the joints previously mentioned, but extremely rare in other joints. This suggests that it is the susceptibility of the joint to the condition that is significant, rather than the transportation through the circulation. (My own) clinical experience suggests that massage does *not* spread the condition to other joints, but such treatment should be given cautiously and the effects carefully monitored.

In remission, the musculature should be treated in the same way as for OA. The joint itself can be treated, but again there is the possibility of causing exacerbation, so initial treatment should be cautious and the results monitored. Friction applied to the soft tissues around the joint can loosen any fibrous adhesions as well as improving the viscosity of joint fluids, and so improve mobility. As there may be a risk of causing inflammation, it may be a good precaution to apply an ice pack immediately after treatment.

The most serious or advanced arthritic conditions can lead to permanent disability, with patients confined to a wheelchair or perhaps unable to use a hand. This presents other massage considerations, which are discussed later (see p.262).

Ankylosing spondylitis This is a progressive inflammatory disease, which seems to be similar to RA and affects the sacroiliac, spinal and costovertebral joints. Inflammation usually starts at the sacroiliac joint and eventually spreads to the surrounding tissues and joints. The chronic inflammation leads to fibrosis, which calcifies and eventually ossifies the bones together, which, of course, affects the musculature.

Inflammation is usually mild but fairly continuous, and so layers of fibrous tissue keep forming. Deep friction massage can loosen this and, combined with correct exercise, means that the thickening fibres form along the lines of stress and therefore do not cause as much dysfunction. General deep massage throughout the lower back and hip muscles will prevent the areas from stiffening up and will encourage better movement, so providing less chance for the bones to fuse together.

Prolapsed invertebral disc

Although this is a condition commonly called a 'slipped disc', it is not possible for a disc to actually slip. The intervertebral disc is made up of two parts, the inside being a soft, very elastic gel and the outside comprising fibrous tissue and fibro cartilage, which is much firmer. Excessive compression on a specific part of the outer ring, such as when picking up a heavy load when the spine is bent, can cause localized damage. The soft jelly inside can seep out and create a protrusion on the outside of the disc, which can affect other structures such as a nerve (causing neuralgia).

This can cause acute pain and many of the back muscles, and sometimes the abdomen too, may go into a protective spasm to prevent any movement that would further aggravate the problem. This gives the patient no option but to rest, and indeed that is just what is necessary for initial recovery. The degree of muscle spasm, however, tends to be very great, and even when lying still and flat there may still be considerable discomfort. And the muscle spasm may restrict circulation and therefore slow down recovery.

As intelligent animals, humans can voluntarily take rest without the need to be forced into it by this degree of protective spasm. Providing the patient follows the advice to rest, it is safe to use massage to release muscle spasm and tension, which can ease the patient's discomfort and promote recovery.

The comfort of the patient is extremely important when giving massage and it is usually necessary to place a cushion under the hips when lying prone, or to use a side-lying/hip-flexed position. After the session the patient must carefully be assisted off the couch so that his back muscles stay relaxed; any sudden contraction could put the muscles back into spasm.

Post-operative massage (musculoskeletal)

Surgery may be carried out on a wide variety of musculoskeletal problems, and to deal with all these individually here would be impossible. The principles of treatment outlined here are therefore very general, and it is essential that the therapist discovers as much as possible about any individual situation before deciding if, or how, to proceed. It is necessary to understand the purpose of the operation, which structures were repaired, removed or replaced, and what other tissues may have been disturbed when this was carried out.

In the post-operative stage massage should, in most cases, be an integral part of the rehabilitation programme and the therapist should work under the direction and approval of the supervising practitioner.

If the operation has been a success, with no complications, and the patient is healthy and recovering well, careful massage treatment can often begin within four or five days.

Such early treatment requires great care, and surgical dressings should not be removed as the scar must be kept sterile. It is vital at this stage not to disturb the site of the suture, as this could prevent the fibres knitting together properly. This can be done by covering the area with a towel and applying a light but firm, static pressure a short distance away from it (in a proximal direction). This prevents any movement of the affected tissues, so treatment should cause no discomfort. Use the other hand to apply long strokes and squeezing techniques to the tissues, working from the fixed hand away from the injury (towards the heart) to help reduce the swelling and pressure, and to promote healing through improved circulation. At all times the injured part should be comfortably supported in a neutral, pain-free position or one fixed by the surgeon.

After about a week it should be possible to work closer to the suture. It is a good idea to look at the condition of the scar to make sure that it is healing well and also to see its exact location. To do this, partly remove the dressing but make sure that it is kept clean and that no oil contacts the scar, which must remain dry. Keeping the area sterile is of vital importance and every precaution must be taken. Replace the dressing and cover with a towel. Gently apply light pressure on either side of the suture and draw the skin together slightly. With the scar held together in this way, short gliding strokes in longitudinal and transverse directions can be applied without affecting the scar itself. This can help prevent adhesions forming between the subcutaneous layers, and can stimulate the circulation to promote healing. If any pain is experienced when doing this, do not proceed.

As time goes on, these techniques can be gradually applied more deeply to prevent adhesions forming between underlying structures. After about four weeks, if dressings have been removed and functional exercises have been recommended, normal massage techniques can be used. Gentle friction can be applied around the area and particularly under the scar. This is best done without oil so that the fingers can keep a good grip with the skin, directly adjacent to the scar. Pressure can be applied and then transverse strokes can be made into the tissues beneath the scar.

The need for rest and difficulty in movement during the initial stage of recovery will result in muscle weakness. Often patients will also have had dysfunction for some time before their operation, so this may have become quite considerable. Massage techniques applied to the muscles to release tension and improve tone can assist the effectiveness of the rehabilitation exercises.

Massage treatment can also be of great benefit in many 'medical' post-operative situations by helping to restore the condition of the tissues and promote healing. This should only be done, however, under the direction and approval of the surgeon.

Pre- and post-joint manipulation

In most situations a manipulative therapist (osteopath, chiropractor or physiotherapist) should treat the soft tissues with massage before and after manipulating joints. A massage therapist, who is able to concentrate more time on this soft tissue work, may often be able to do a better and more thorough job.

It is common for a patient to struggle with a problem for a long time before seeking treatment. During this time secondary areas of tension may build up as they compensate for the problem. General massage can help release some of this first, so that the manipulative therapist is better able to assess the root cause of the problem and is not confused by secondary factors. As the tissues are more relaxed, manipulation is also easier to perform and more effective.

After manipulation (up to a few days later) deep massage helps the muscles adjust to the corrected bone alignment and often produces quicker results than manipulation on its own.

Pregnancy

Although pregnancy is not perhaps a medical condition that requires treatment, massage can help to alleviate some of the uncomfortable symptoms that women often get when pregnant. Swelling in the lower legs can be reduced with massage, which can also be used to relieve lower backache.

There are practical problems, as it is not possible to lie the patient in a prone position during the later months. The woman can put herself into a comfortable side-lying position on the couch, and then the therapist can work from the side to treat one side of the back. Then the patient can roll over to allow the other side to be treated. Legs can be treated in the supine position or side-lying.

An alternative method involves the woman sitting on a stool and resting her head and shoulders on a cushion on a table in front of her. The therapist can sit behind her to treat. Although treating pregnant women may present some physical difficulties to the therapist, it can be well worth the effort.

Severe disability and terminal disease

This is a very special area of work for the massage therapist to experience. Without the goals of treating and improving a condition, we must be able to see the great value in simply enhancing the quality and dignity of human life, at whatever level. This type of work requires a highly individual approach, looking at the particular strengths and weaknesses as well as the general, physical and emotional needs of the patient. Their likes and dislikes of particular massage techniques should also be considered, so that they get the most benefit and enjoyment out of the treatment.

The psychological effects of massage can sometimes be the most significant part of the treatment, although these are rarely mentioned or recognized. Touch and feel are very important senses, which add much to our quality of life but are taken for granted by normal healthy people. Many severely ill and disabled people may not be able to reach out and touch, and may only feel touch when being 'handled' during clinical or nursing procedures. Massage is a sensual experience that they can enjoy, and this should be seen as an important and valid aspect of treatment.

Communicating well with the patient can also enhance the treatment. Physical disability and illness do not necessarily affect a person's mind, but all too often patients are spoken to like children and the massage therapist must not make this mistake. Treatment takes time, and talking and working at the same time are easy, so make it a friendly visit.

Severely ill or disabled people need as much help as possible, and even with the best medical care there is always room for something more. The medical teams working in these areas are usually very willing to give advice and guidance on how the massage therapist can help improve the quality of the patient's life.

Disability When use of a part of the body has been permanently lost, the patient must develop means of compensating by using the rest of his body in different ways to help him live as normal a life as possible. This means that some areas will need to develop more strength or flexibility, and could therefore become over-used or eventually suffer from arthritic changes. With advanced knowledge of these potential problems, preventative massage treatment can be given to maintain healthy function in these areas.

Loss of movement leads to muscle wastage and a slow-down in circulation, which can cause general aching and discomfort, and massage to the affected limb will help maintain its general health and prevent this. If the patient is confined to a wheelchair (or bed), the problem can be more general, affecting the circulation in the whole body. Although a full general massage to the whole body may be a good idea, it is often impractical, as undressing and getting onto a couch can take the patient a lot of time and effort. Working through clothes and treating a patient in the wheelchair or bed may be uncomfortable for the therapist, but that just has to be accepted. Simply squeezing the tissues will have a pumping effect on the circulation, but this can be enhanced by using the elasticity of the skin to make a stroke towards the heart while squeezing.

Long periods of sitting put pressure on the buttock and hamstring muscles, which restricts circulation and can affect the sciatic nerve. If possible, slide a hand under the buttocks and apply squeezing and rotation movements. Although this may look rather peculiar, it can ease much discomfort and relieve pressure.

Staying in a fixed position with the joints flexed, as when sitting, eventually leads to permanent contracture (shortening) of the flexor muscles, such as the ilia/psoas and hamstrings, which do not get stretched. These contractures add to the disability as they stop full extension of the joints, which can prevent even a normal comfortable sleeping position in bed. Passive stretching to the contracted muscles and strengthening exercises (if possible) to the antagonist muscles can help prevent this problem.

Terminal disease   There are, sadly, many terminal illnesses, all of which have their own characteristics, and each patient may have his or her own unique pattern of symptoms. The therapist must discover as much as possible about the nature and development of the particular disease and, wherever possible, must try to ease the symptoms and delay the onset of future symptoms. With diseases like cancer it can be argued that massage may spread it to other areas, but if it has been diagnosed as 'terminal', then it is perhaps right to offer the help that massage may provide and let the patient decide.

The powerful medication often given to the terminally ill can have strong side-effects, which in some cases can be anticipated and possibly prevented. For instance, patients with multiple sclerosis are sometimes injected with large doses of steroids, which can cause necrosis (starvation of blood) to the hip joint as a side-effect. Plenty of deep petrissage around the joint will help prevent this. The long-term use of oral medication, and constant compression of the viscera due to sitting, can lead to digestion problems including constipation, which can also usefully be helped by massage.

There are too many conditions to list here, and treatments should always be unique to the individual. The following are just two examples, which will hopefully provide some ideas on how to approach all such situations.

Multiple sclerosis   This is a degenerative disease of the nervous system, which is possibly caused by the auto-immune system and affects the myelin sheath surrounding the nerves. Symptoms affect motor function first, with both muscle wastage and atrophy in some muscles, and spasm and hypertrophy (spasticity) in other muscles. There are also involuntary movements that cause patients to stumble and fall quite often, which can lead to other injuries. The condition tends to develop with periods of exacerbation and remission.

The muscular symptoms can be treated as they develop and change. Tight muscles can be stretched with deep stroking massage and passive stretching (unless this causes the muscle to go into spasm). Weak areas can be treated to improve tone and can be strengthened with active and resisted exercises up to maximal strength (but the patient should not become generally fatigued by the exercises).

Exercise is vital to help prevent the development of the disease, and the therapist must encourage the patient to persevere with this. As the symptoms change, the therapist can give regular advice on specific areas that must be strengthened or stretched.

Vigorous tapotement techniques can stimulate the nervous system and many patients seem to find it extremely helpful. The benefits to weak muscles are good, although it could cause spasm in hyper-tense areas, so the patient should decide how they would like it used.

Muscular dystrophy This is a hereditary, degenerative disease that affects all the muscles, and it is usually boys who are afflicted with it. There is no known cure or even medication to delay its progress, and screening during pregnancy is the only preventative measure available at the present time. By early teens the boy's disability is already quite severe, he will usually be confined to a wheelchair and will rarely survive beyond 20 years.

The purpose of treatment can only be to enhance the comfort of the patient and provide friendly support. General stiffness, aching and discomfort through lack of activity are a constant problem. Rubbing and squeezing techniques, as well as passive movements, will help blood-flow and so ease these. Pressure on the sciatic nerve due to a combination of muscle wastage in the buttocks and long periods of sitting can be helped with treatment in this area, too.

Contractures are a major problem, as all flexor muscles will shorten, adding the problem of severe joint restriction to the muscle wasting. Active and resisted exercises to the extensor muscles can be tried to help prevent wastage, but the effects are only minimal. Passive stretching to the contracted flexors will help and should be done as often as possible (advise the patient's carers to do this daily, if possible). Contractures in the elbows and hands need the most attention, as these will be the last important tools that the patient will have.

Long periods of sitting and lack of muscular support cause the patient to squash down in his chair, and after a few years of this a severe scoliosis (sideways bend) in the spine will develop. This leads to a crease forming in the side of the body, as the ribs and pelvis gradually move together on one side. The soft tissues in this area become very congested and uncomfortable. One way to help ease this discomfort is to put the patient on his side (creased side up), making sure he is well supported with cushions. Squeezing techniques can be applied into the crease and along the back to promote circulation. Also, in this position the crease can be stretched out by gently pushing the hip and lower ribs away from each other.

18 Self-Massage

Self-massage is the most natural form of therapy, which is instinctively understood by most people from their very early childhood. It takes little instruction by the therapist to enable the patient to apply self-massage to help deal with his own minor injuries. This can continue the benefits of treatment and so greatly improve recovery time.

Sportsmen can be instructed to use self-massage on a regular basis to help promote recovery after hard exercise. Therapists should also set a good example and use it for their own injuries, especially over-use problems in the hands and arms.

There are limitations to self-massage, as it is rarely possible to apply the same pressure or to use the same variety of techniques. But it can still have the same basic benefits as massage treatment in the clinical environment.

The key to successful self-massage is to ensure that the muscle being treated is in a shortened and relaxed position. This means that a different body position is needed for each part. The following examples show just a few possibilities, but with practice and experience these can be developed to give a very thorough and effective overall treatment.

Calf muscles: resting the leg through the heel so that the foot is plantaflexed, which shortens and relaxes the muscles. The hands can squeeze and stroke up the group with deep friction and stroking applied where necessary.

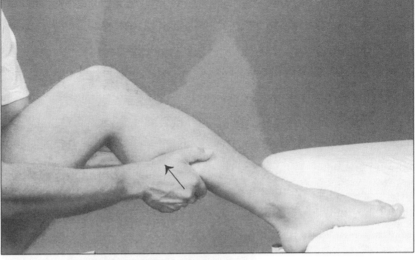

Calf muscles: resting the leg through the outside of the foot makes it possible to use kneading techniques. This is also a good position from which to apply deep friction with the thumb.

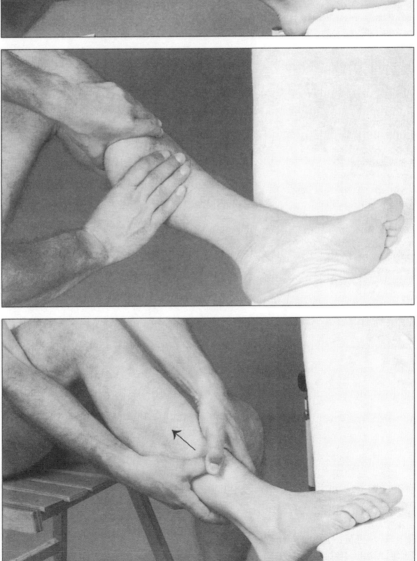

Anterior and lateral muscles: resting through the inside of the foot offers good access to the lateral muscles. Deep pressure can be applied with the thumbs and the stroke is made by pulling up the leg. To treat the tibialis anterior the same method is used, but with the leg resting through the forefoot.

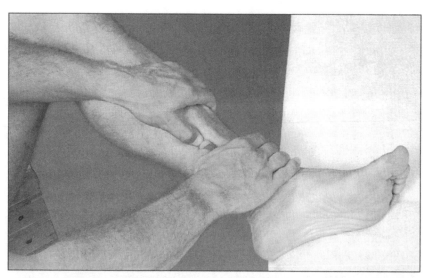

Shin: resting through the lateral ankle, with the hip abducted and outwardly rotated and the knee flexed. In this position deep friction and stroking can be applied with the thumbs along the medial tibial border. This is very beneficial in treating or preventing 'shin splints'.

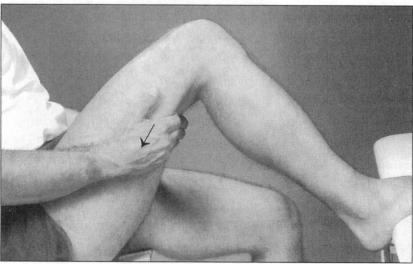

Hamstrings: with the weight of the leg supported and the knee flexed at about 90 degrees. The fingers can curl deep into the muscles as strokes are applied from the knee to the buttocks. The stroke can stop where necessary to apply friction and transverse stroking, by rocking the fingers from side to side.

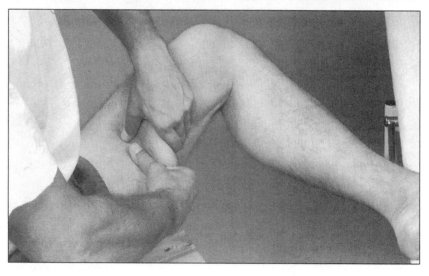

Adductors: with the leg turned out and the knee flexed, by twisting the trunk towards the other leg it is possible to apply kneading and stroking techniques.

Quadriceps: with the leg resting in extension, the back must be supported in an upright position to prevent any active hip flexion, which would not allow the group to relax fully. Both hands can press down into the muscles and pull back to make the stroke.

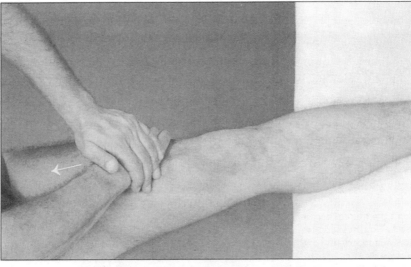

Quadriceps: with the torso turned towards the treated leg, kneading techniques can be applied.

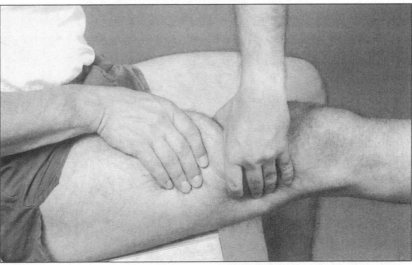

Iliotibial band (example: right leg): with the leg extended, the heel of the right palm applies the stroke by pulling up the leg, while the left hand comes across and pulls it into the tissues to increase the pressure.

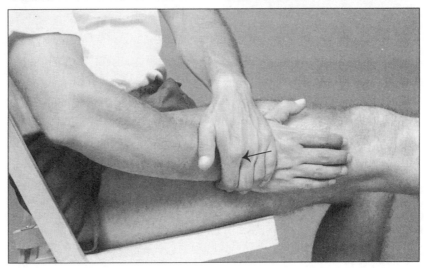

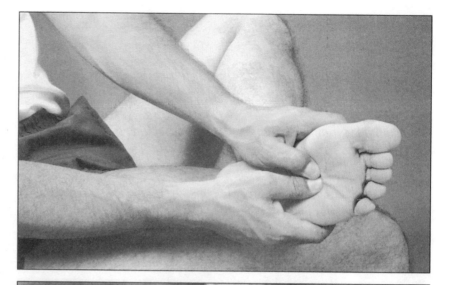

Foot: the thumbs can be used all over the foot to apply deep stroking and friction.

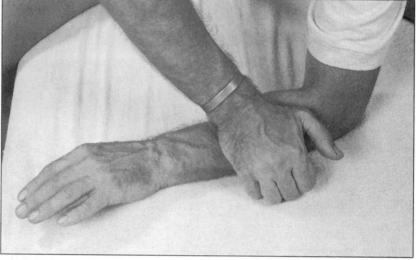

Forearm: with one arm resting on a table, the heel of the other palm can be used to apply deep pressure and stroking techniques.

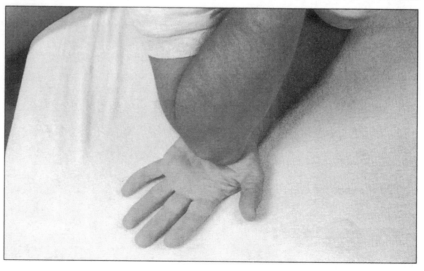

Palm: with the hand resting out flat, the elbow of the other arm can be used for deep friction into the muscles. For lighter techniques, simply use one hand to treat the other.

'Tennis elbow': using an STR technique, with the arm hanging down and the elbow locked in full extension by contracting the triceps. The fingers of the other hand are pressed firmly into the affected tissues and this hand is also used to shake the whole arm. With the wrist held loose, there will be considerable joint movement, as it swings when the arm is shaken. This creates the stretch on the muscle, which is focused into the affected tissues by the applied pressure.

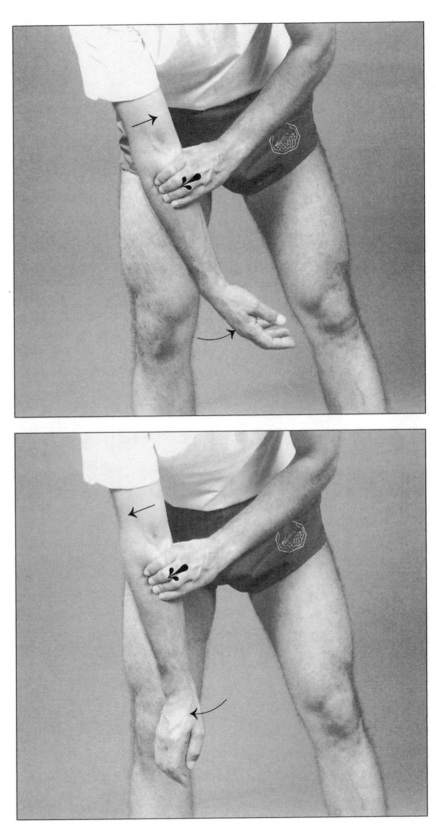

Appendix 1

Structure and function of the musculoskeletal soft tissues

Brief descriptions

Bursa

A sac-like structure filled with fluid (similar to synovial fluid). It is found between different tissue structures, usually around a joint, and acts to prevent friction between them as they move. With a soft fluid centre, it also acts as a cushion to absorb shock.

Small pads of fat (fat-pads) can also form between tissues around a joint, or at other sites subject to external pressure or rubbing. They fulfil much the same function as a bursa.

Cartilage

Articular cartilage is a dense layer of connective tissue, which covers the articulating surfaces of a bone, inside the synovial capsule. It provides a smooth surface so that the bones can glide without friction.

Some joints contain pads, or discs, of fibro cartilage, which fill the spaces between the articular surfaces and provide them with a good fitting. They can also help to absorb shock (menisci of the knee and elbow, and intervertebral discs).

Ligament

A tough band of fibrous tissue that links bones together across a joint. The fibres run in parallel and in line with the direction of stress. A ligament is inelastic but flexible, so it allows free movement within a certain range, but restricts any movement beyond it, which might otherwise result in bone damage. It therefore supports and protects the joint.

It has a relatively poor blood supply and takes longer to heal than muscle.

Muscle

A muscle is composed of many thousands of fibres, which lie in parallel and are bound together into small bundles by connective tissue. These bundles are contained within compartments that together form the whole muscle, which is surrounded in a fascial sheath of connective tissue.

Each fibre is supplied by a nerve which, when stimulated, can cause a rapid contraction. The individual fibres contract on an all-or-nothing principle, so if the muscle as a whole is contracting at 50 per cent of its strength, then 50 per cent of the fibres are fully contracting. If the effort is sustained, the contracting fibres fatigue and, as they relax, the resting fibres are recruited to take up the effort.

A muscle is only able to contract or relax. By attaching to a bone (via tendons) across a joint, the contraction shortens the muscle and so creates articular movement.

Muscles have a rich blood supply and tend to heal quickly after injury.

Synovial (articular) capsule

Some joints are referred to as synovial, or a freely movable joint. The joint cavity is enclosed in a capsule made by a synovial membrane, which is a loose and fairly elastic connective tissue. This secretes synovial fluid, which fills the capsule, and lubricates and nourishes the inner joint structures, especially the articular cartilage.

Tendon

A tough cord made up of parallel bundles of collagen fibres, which extend from the connective tissue surrounding the muscle and its compartments. It attaches the muscle at one end to the bone, via the periosteum at the other end. Although often considered to be inflexible, it can actually accommodate about 5 per cent of stretch, which enables it to absorb the shock of a sudden forced contraction. Its relative inflexibility transmits the force of contraction from the muscle to the bone so that movement takes place.

Appendix 2

Location and directional terms

Medial:	Towards the centre, or midline of the body
Lateral:	Towards the outer side, or away from the midline of the body
Anterior:	Towards the front of the body
Posterior:	Towards the back of the body
Superior:	Above, or towards the top of the body
Inferior:	Below, or towards the bottom of the body
Proximal:	Towards the centre of the body, or another structure
Distal:	Away from the centre of the body, or another structure.
Peripheral:	Towards the surface of the body
Palmar:	On or towards the palm of the hand
Plantar:	On or towards the sole of the foot
Dorsal:	Towards the back of the body (or back of the hand, top of the foot)
Cranial:	Towards the head
Caudal:	Towards the buttocks
Ventral:	Towards the abdomen
Longitudinal:	Vertical, when the body is in an upright position. In line with the fibres, when referring to a particular area of tissue.
Transverse:	Horizontal across the body. Across the fibres, when referring to a particular area of tissue.
Internal or inward:	Turning in towards the midline (as seen from the front of the body).
External or outward:	Turning out from the midline.

Appendix 3

Movements

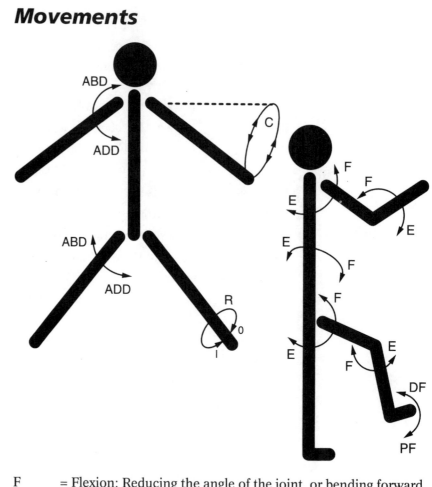

F	= Flexion: Reducing the angle of the joint, or bending forward
E	= Extension: Increasing the angle of the joint, or leaning back
DF/PF	= Dorsiflexion and plantaflexion, when referring to the foot
ABD	= Abduction: Moving away from the midline of the body
ADD	= Adduction: Moving toward the midline of the body
C	= Circumduction: A circular movement
R	= Rotation: A rotary or pivoting movement
.I	= Internal/inward
O	= Outward/external

Others (not shown on Figures)

Lateral flexion:	Side-bending the trunk
Elevation:	Drawn upwards
Depression:	Drawn downwards
Protraction:	Drawn forward
Retraction:	Drawn backward (with the scapula this is also adduction)
Pronation:	Rotating the forearm with the palm turning inwards
Supination:	Rotating the arm with the palm turning outwards
Radial flexion (adduction):	With the palm facing forward, the hand moves, from the wrist, away from the body
Ulna flexion (adduction):	As above, but moves towards the body
Eversion (pronation):	Forefoot moves away from the body and the sole turns outwards
Inversion (supination):	Forefoot moves towards the body and the sole turns inwards

Joints

Ball-and-socket joint
Movements: Flexion/extension, adduction/abduction, circumduction and rotation
A rounded head of a bone fits into a cup-shaped cavity, enabling movement in all planes.

Condyloid and saddle joints
Movements: Flexion/extension, adduction/abduction, some circumduction
Where convex and concave surfaces join along a curve or saddle, allowing movement in two planes.

Gliding joint
Movement: Gliding
Two flat surfaces that glide over each other.

Hinge joint
Movement: Flexion and extension
A convex surface fitting into a concave surface, which allows movement in one plane only.

Pivot joint
Movement: Rotation
A socket in one bone rotating around a peg on another.

Joint	Type
Atlas and axis:	Pivot
Inter vertebrae:	Gliding
Vertebra and rib:	Gliding
Costal cartilage and sternum:	Gliding
Sternum and clavicle (sternoclavicular):	Gliding, with disc of cartilage
Clavicle and scapula (acromioclavicular):	Gliding, with slight rotation
Scapula and humerus (glenohumeral):	Ball-and-socket
Humerus and ulna:	Hinge
Humerus and radius:	Hinge, and rotation
Radius (head) and ulna:	Gliding/pivot
Radius and ulna (distal):	Gliding/pivot
Radius, ulna and carpals (wrist):	Condyloid
Carpal joints:	Gliding
Trapezium and metacarpal (thumb):	Saddle
Carpals and metacarpals:	Gliding
Metacarpals and phalanges:	Condyloid
Phalanges (fingers):	Hinge
Ilium and sacrum (sacroiliac):	Gliding, with only limited movement
Acetabulum and femur (hip):	Ball-and-socket
Femur and tibia:	Structurally condyloid but functionally a hinge joint with semi-lunar cartilages
Femur and patella:	Gliding
Tibia and fibula (head):	Gliding
Tibia, fibula and talus (ankle):	Hinge
Tarsal joints:	Gliding
Tarsals and metatarsals:	Gliding
Metatarsals and phalanges:	Condyloid
Phalanges (toes):	Hinge

Bibliography

General Anatomical Chart Co., Chicago: *Muscular and Skeletal Systems*
Brukner, P., Khan, K.: *Clinical Sports Medicine*, McGraw-Hill, 1993
Butler, D.: *Mobilisation of the Nervous System*, Churchill Livingstone, 1991
Chaitow, L.: *Soft Tissue Manipulation*, Thorsons, 1980
Chaitow, L.: *Osteopathic Self Treatment*, Thorsons, 1990
Chaitow, L.: *Palpatory Literacy*, Thorsons, 1991
Ebner, M.: *Connective Tissue Manipulation*, Robert E. Krieger, 1985
Feldenkrais, M.: *Awareness Through Movement*, Penguin, 1972
Hemery, D., Ogden, G., Evans, A.: *Winning Without Drugs*, Collins Willow, 1990
McMinn, R., Hutchings, R.: *A Colour Atlas of Human Anatomy*, 2nd ed., Wolfe Medical, 1988
Newton, J., Durkin, F.: *Running to the Top of the Mountain*, J. & J. Winning Edge, 1988
Noakes, T.: *Lore of Running*, Leisure Press, 1991
Peterson, L., Renstrom, P.: *Sports Injuries, Their Prevention and Treatment*, Dunitz, 1986
Platzer, W.: *Color Atlas and Textbook of Human Anatomy*, vol. 1: Locomotor System, Georg Thieme Verlag, 1986
Read, M., Wade, P.: *Sports Injuries*, Breslich & Foss, 1984
Rees, P., Williams, D.: *Principles of Clinical Medicine*, Edward Arnold, 1995
Rowett, H.: *Basic Anatomy and Physiology*, 2nd ed., John Murray, 1973
Southmayd, W., Marshall, H.: *Sports Health*, Putnam, 1981
Stirk, J: *Structural Fitness*, Elm Tree, 1988
Stone, R., Stone, J.; *Atlas of the Skeletal Muscles*, Wm C. Brown, 1990
Subotnick, S.: *Sport and Exercise Injuries*, North Atlantic Books, 1991
Thompson, A., Skinner, A., Piercy, J.: *Tidy's Physiotherapy*,12th ed., Butterworth Heinemann, 1991
Tortora, G.: *Introduction to the Human Body*, 2nd ed., Harper Collins, 1991

Voss, D., Ionta, M., Myers, B.: *Proprioceptive Neuromuscular Facilitation,* 3rd ed., Harper & Row, 1985

Wale, J.: *Tidy's Massage and Remedial Exercises,* 11th ed., John Wright & Son, 1968

Wirhed, R.: *Athletic Ability and the Anatomy of Motion*, Wolfe Medical, 1984

Wood & Becker: *Beard's Massage,* 3rd ed., W. B. Saunders, 1964

Ylinen, J., Cash, M.: *Sports Massage*, Stanley Paul, 1988

Acupressure   Kaptchuk, Ted J.: *Chinese Medicine: The Web That Has No Weaver*, Rider, 1983

Low, Royston: *The Acupuncture Atlas and Reference Book*, Thorsons, 1985

Jarmey, C., Tindall, J.: *Acupressure for Common Ailments*, Gaia, 1991

General index

Index of muscles